CARDIOLOGY

SERVET
CLINICAL GUIDE

CHRONIC VALVULAR DISEASE

Joaquín Bernal de Pablo-Blanco

Plaza Antonio Beltrán Martínez nº 1, planta 8 - letra I
(Centro empresarial El Trovador)
50002 Zaragoza - Spain

First printing: April 2019

This book was originally published in Spanish under the title:
Guía servet de manejo clínico. Endocardiosis valvular crónica
© 2018 Grupo Asís Biomedia, SL
ISBN Spanish edition: 978-84-17225-64-3

Translation:
Lori Newman

ISBN: 978-84-17640-00-2
DL: Z 688-2019

Design, layout and printing:
Servet editorial - Grupo Asís Biomedia, SL
www.grupoasis.com
info@grupoasis.com

GRUPO asis

Servet is the publishing house of Grupo Asís

Warning:

Veterinary science is constantly evolving, as are pharmacology and the other sciences. Inevitably, it is therefore the responsibility of the veterinary surgeon to determine and verify the dosage, the method of administration, the duration of treatment and any possible contraindications to the treatments given to each individual patient, based on his or her professional experience. Neither the publisher nor the author can be held liable for any damage or harm caused to people, animals or properties resulting from the correct or incorrect application of the information contained in this book.

ACKNOWLEDGEMENTS

"People are most likely to believe what they least understand."
Michel de Montaigne (1533–1592)

Thank you to the whole Servet team for trusting me once more and believing in these guides designed to assist in managing the most common diseases of companion animals.

I would especially like to thank the design team, Mercedes González for her marketing efforts, and project managers Yolanda Vela and Leticia Escuín for their unwavering support.

I am also grateful to all the entrepreneurs in the veterinary sector whose initiatives enable a miraculous symbiosis between clinicians, researchers, and communication networks towards the goals of converting a molecule into a commercial drug for clinical use and sharing the information to benefit all stakeholders – patients, pet owners, and veterinary surgeons.

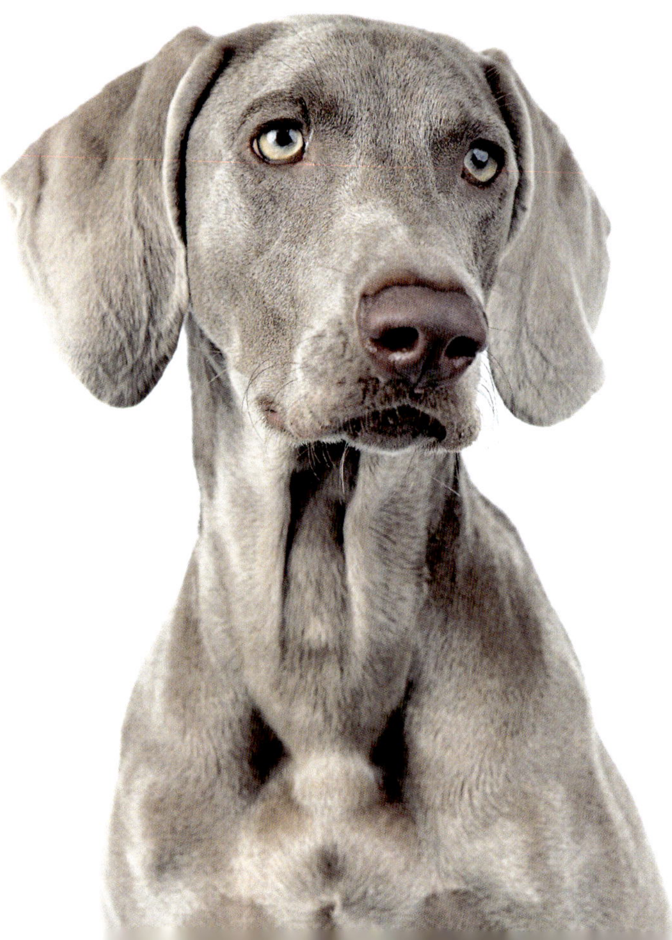

THE AUTHOR

JOAQUÍN BERNAL DE PABLO-BLANCO

He graduated in veterinary medicine from the Complutense University of Madrid (Spain) and completed a postgraduate course at the Animal Medical Center of New York (USA).

He is a member and former vice-president of the Cardiology and Respiratory Specialists Group (GECAR) of the Spanish Small Animal Veterinary Association (AVEPA) and a member of the European Society of Veterinary Cardiology (ESVC).

He has practised solely veterinary cardiology since 1995.

He is a founding partner and director of Cardiovet, an international telediagnostic cardiology and respiratory referral service for veterinary practices in Spain, Portugal, and Latin America.

Since 2003, he has been a principal investigator and consultant in electrocardiography and telemetry analysis in preclinical toxicology, pharmacodynamics, and pharmaceutical safety studies for human and veterinary drug development (CIDA SAL, Harlan, Vivotecnia). He is currently engaged in scientific research at the centres Envigo Spain and Envigo UK.

He is the author and coauthor of several books and dozens of articles on cardiology, electrocardiography, and related topics, as well as a frequent lecturer on these topics at live seminars and online courses both in Spain and internationally.

FOREWORD

When we first thought of establishing an electrocardiography interpretation service, back in the 20th century, our goal was to help clinicians inexperienced in cardiology to interpret electrocardiograms; that is, to count squares, measure, label, and name the patterns on the "strip". It would be an ECG-Spanish/Spanish-ECG translation service.

In those days, an anxious fax from a colleague preoccupied us with a much greater and simpler problem than we had anticipated: "Is there a heart? Help!"

From the inception of that service until today, what most veterinary surgeons have asked us to determine is not the names of the arrhythmias, the heart rate, or whether the P wave equals X or the T-wave is biphasic; instead, their main concern is whether a dog's cough is of cardiac or respiratory origin.

The vast majority of our heart disease patients have chronic valvular disease (CVD). The classic case is an elderly small-breed dog with a cough and exercise intolerance. The problem is that this is also the classic signalment of chronic respiratory disease, with matching clinical signs: cough and dyspnoea. To complicate matters further, many dogs with CVD tend to also present with chronic respiratory disease or even Cushing's disease.

The goal of this guide is to resolve this quandary thoroughly and accurately while remaining faithful to real clinical practice. This guide avoids contrived and overly academic language and offers solutions for all clinicians, regardless of their experience in the field or their technical capabilities.

Chronic valvular disease appears routinely in the clinic, so I hope the reader finds this guide useful and practical for managing this disease safely, effectively, and confidently.

Enrique Ynaraja
Cardiovet
Albeytar veterinary services

PREFACE

General practice veterinary surgeons often regard cardiologists as specialists who handle extremely complex cases using sophisticated methods and techniques: valvoplasty, doppler echocardiography, tracheal stenting, pacemakers, Holter monitors, closure of patent ductus arteriosus, angiography, etc.

The reality is much less glamourous: 7 or 8 out of every 10 dogs with heart disease have chronic valvular disease (CVD), a degenerative disease that typically affects the mitral valve. The more small, elderly dogs we treat, the more common the disease.

Thus, the mitral valve occupies most of our workday and puts food on the table. Without the disease-prone mitral valve, most cardiologists would be performing skin scrapes in search of elusive mites, and the most “digital” activity of our day would be rectal palpation.

The good news is that to succeed in managing CVD, it is not necessary to take a poodle to Houston, get a degree in "Cor triatriatum and other rare heart diseases" from the University of Pennsylvania, or purchase a non-deductible $25,000 echocardiography machine.

Our friend the stethoscope, a set of chest X-rays, an ECG strip, and a dose of common sense and due diligence are all that is required to manage this disease.

Groucho Marx said, “Politics is the art of finding problems everywhere, misdiagnosing them, and fixing them incorrectly.” I could not agree more with this view, and I always strive to avoid making the kinds of errors he joked about.

As its title suggests, this guide is intended to orient the primary care veterinary surgeon on the correct path for CVD diagnosis and treatment as well as assist in client communication. I hope to have achieved this goal.

The author, Joaquín Bernal
Cardiovet

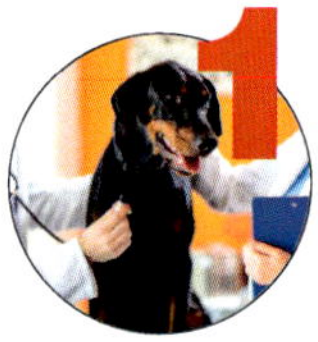

1 READ ME FIRST

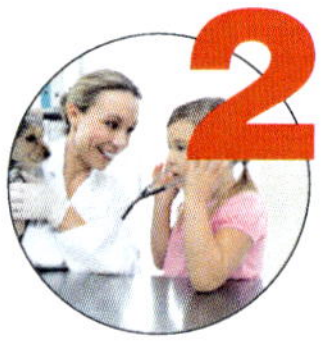

2 AT THE CLINIC

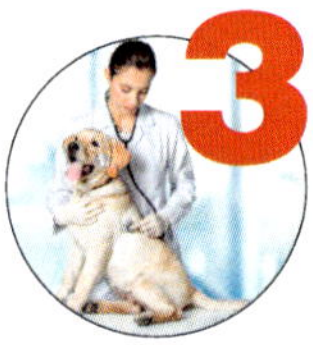

3 DIAGNOSIS

TABLE OF CONTENTS

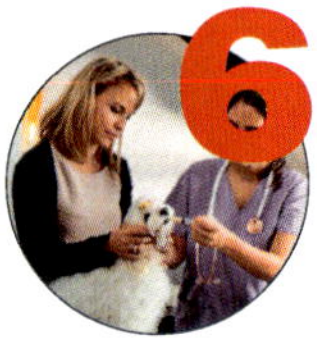

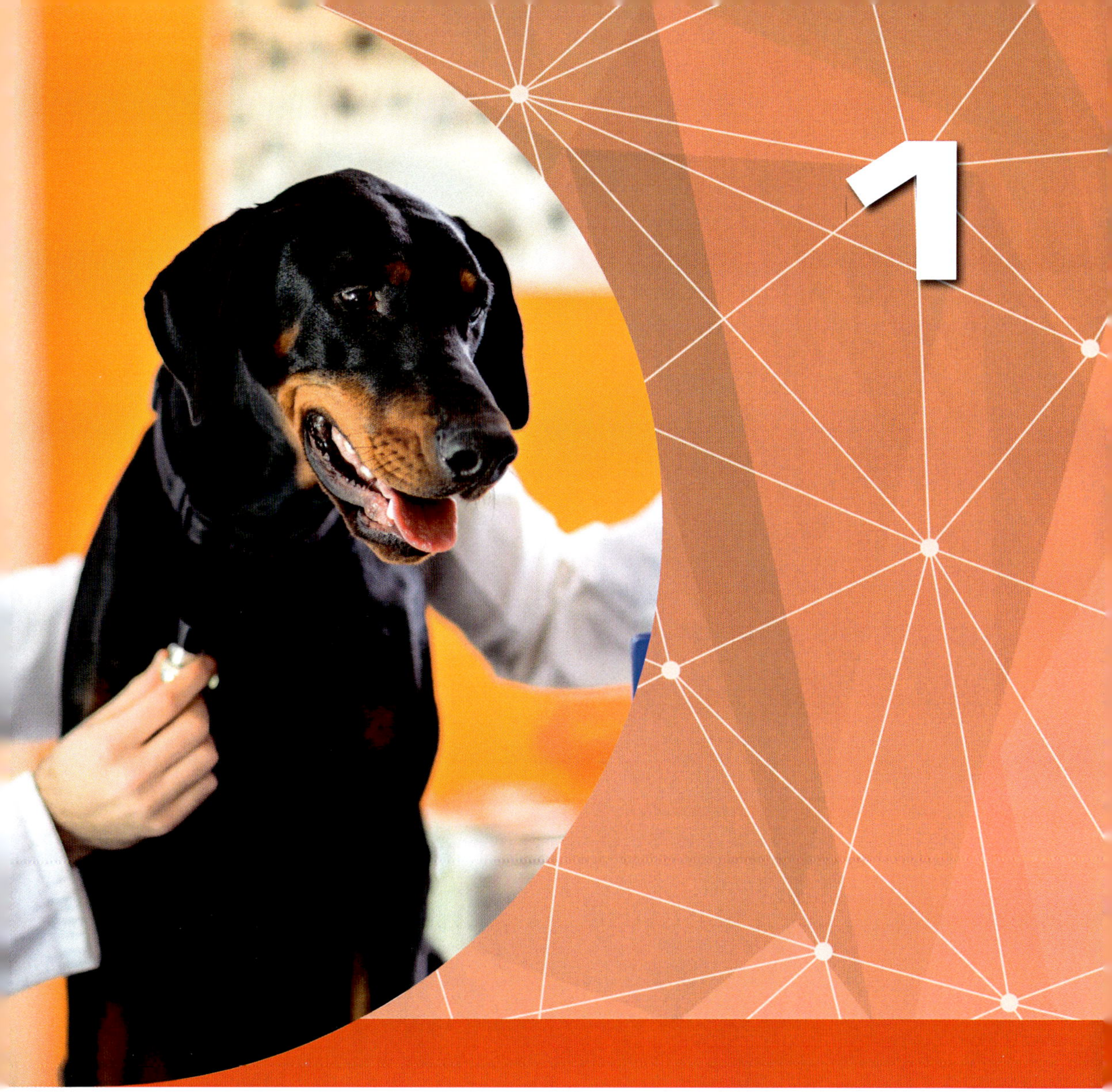

1

READ ME FIRST

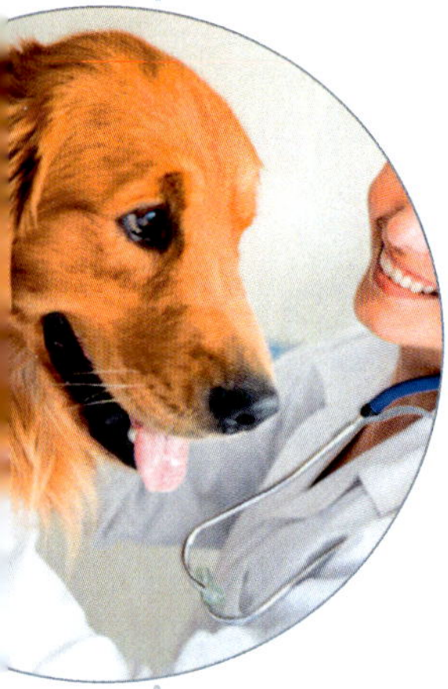

The mitral valve is located between the left atrium and the left ventricle. It allows ventricular filling by opening during diastole and prevents reflux of blood into the left atrium by closing during systole, the interval of ventricular contraction and ejection of blood through the major arteries (the aorta in the case of the left heart) (Fig. 1).

Age-related degeneration of this valve is quite common in dogs and leads to improper valve closure, known as chronic valvular disease (CVD).

MITRAL VALVE ANATOMY

The anatomical structure that regulates blood flow through the mitral orifice is called the mitral apparatus or mitral complex.

Its anatomical components are as follows (Fig. 2):

- Posterior wall of the left atrium.
- Mitral annulus.
- Mitral valve.
- Chordae tendinae.
- Papillary muscles.
- Left ventricular free wall.

Figure 1. FUNCTION OF THE MITRAL VALVE

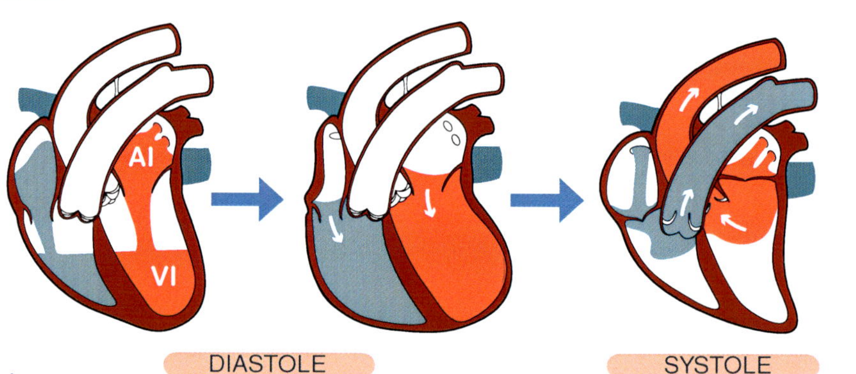

The mitral valve regulates blood flow from the left atrium to the left ventricle. It remains open in diastole to allow ventricular filling and closes in systole to prevent reflux.

The valve leaflets are attached at their base to a fibrous annulus that forms part of the cardiac skeleton. The chordae tendinae insert at the leaflet margins, restricting their movement and ensuring valve closure without leaks.

The papillary muscles, which are muscular projections of the ventricle, form the supports for the chordae.

Mitral valve movement was initially thought to be a passive function of the pressures generated inside the heart. However, the valve opening and closure are now known to be active movements resulting from synchronous motion of all parts of the valve.

Thus, a change in any of these elements can cause mitral insufficiency, but the most common process in dogs is degeneration of the valve itself.

Figure 2 ANATOMY OF THE MITRAL COMPLEX

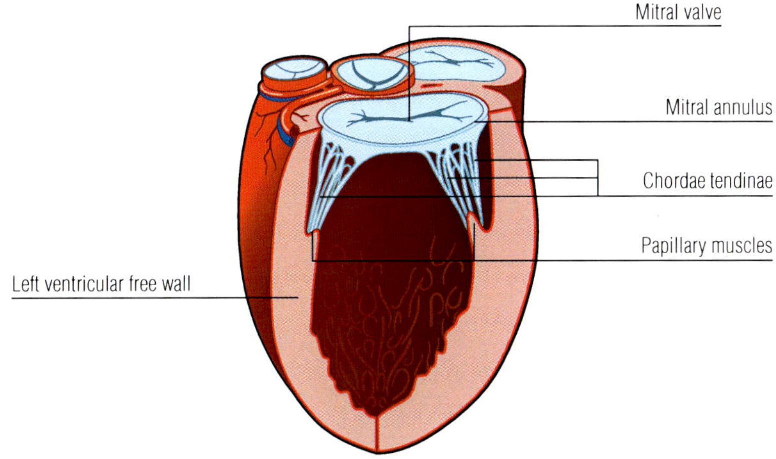

A normal mitral valve contains four distinct histological layers, in order from the atrium to the ventricle (Fig. 3):

- Atrialis layer: continuation of the atrial endocardium.
- Spongiosa layer: collection of scattered fibres and bundles of collagen with some elastic fibres embedded in a mucopolysaccharide material.
- Fibrosa layer: constitutes the valve skeleton. It is made of a dense collagen layer and is continuous with the mitral annulus and chordae tendinae.
- Ventricularis layer: continuation of the ventricular endocardium.

Figure 3 HISTOLOGICAL STRUCTURE OF THE MITRAL VALVE

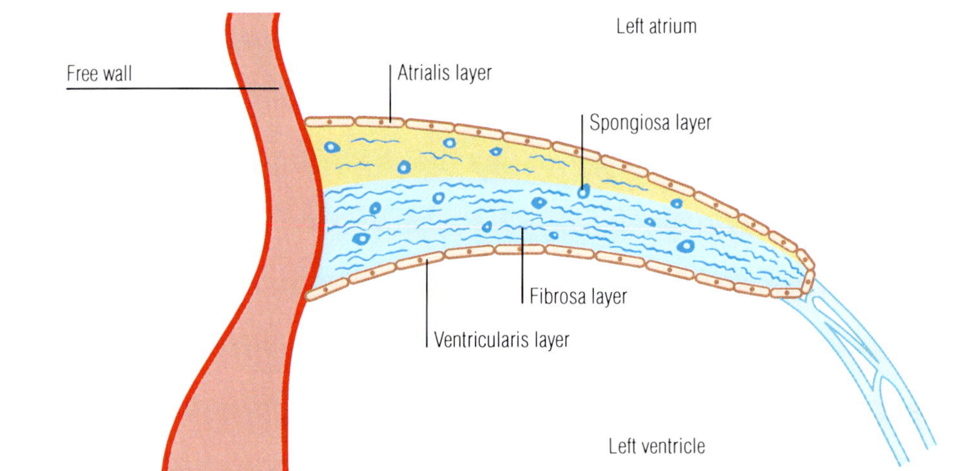

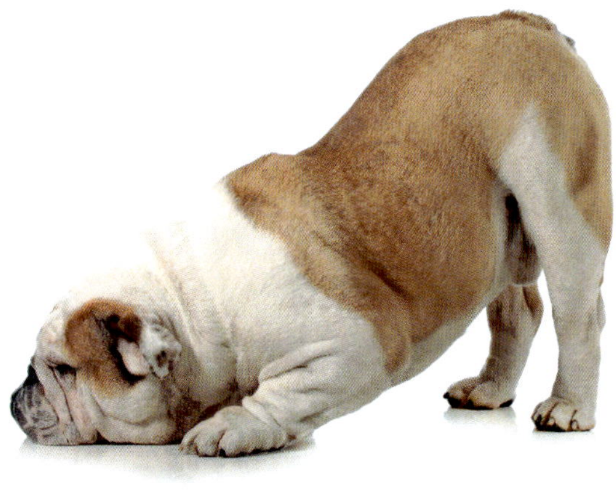

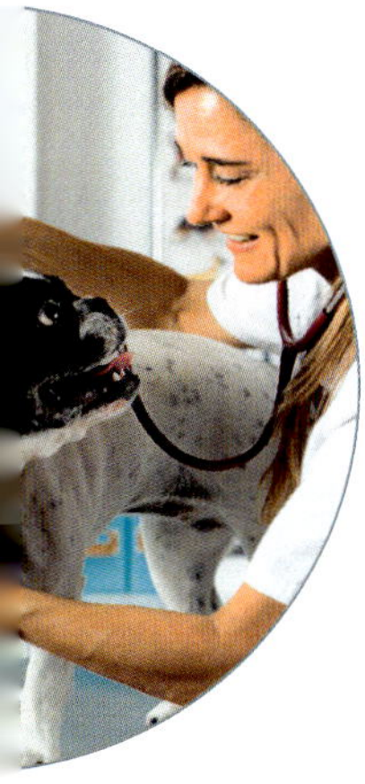

AETIOLOGY
OF CHRONIC VALVULAR DISEASE

The aetiology of this process is unknown. Several theories exist.

Collagen degeneration may be hereditary to some degree, according to studies performed in certain chondrodystrophic breeds predisposed to CVD such as the Cavalier King Charles Spaniel and the Dachshund.

These same breeds often have connective tissue disorders such as intervertebral disc disease, cranial cruciate ligament rupture, dorsal tracheal collapse, and periodontal disease, suggesting a defect in the extracellular matrix.

Several mutations that affect connective tissue have been discovered in human genes for different types of collagen. The histopathological changes associated with those mutations resemble those seen in dogs with mitral degeneration, suggesting that those alterations may be involved in canine CVD.

Certain authors believe that changes in the synthesis, content and organisation of collagen fibres underlie the pathological process of myxomatous degeneration, also called "dyscollagenosis".

Other possible causes include alterations in collagen degradation enzymes.

Other proposed aetiologies include:

- Stress.
- Hypertension.
- Hypoxia.
- Viral or bacterial infections.
- Several endocrine disorders.

However, no clear links between CVD and bacterial infections or immune-mediated processes have been found; some authors advocate a relationship between CVD and hyperadrenocorticism because some studies have reproduced valvular lesions in patients under stress that resemble those of spontaneous CVD. While the cause remains unknown, chronic valvular disease is considered a non-infectious, non-inflammatory degenerative process.

WHAT IS
CHRONIC VALVULAR DISEASE?

Chronic valvular disease is also referred to as the following:

- Chronic atrioventricular valve endocardiosis.
- Chronic valvular insufficiency.
- Chronic valvular fibrosis.
- Age-related valvular endocardiosis.
- Myxomatous valvular degeneration.

Figure 4

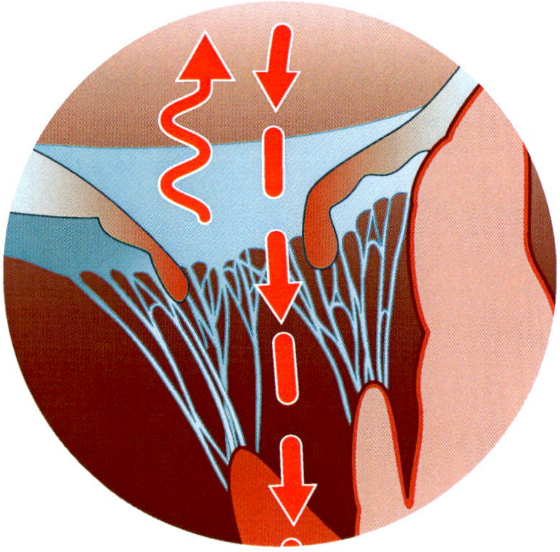

Degeneration of the mitral valve prevents its closure during systole and allows blood regurgitation into the left atrium.

The mitral valve should remain completely closed during systole to prevent regurgitation of blood into the left atrium. Myxomatous degeneration of the valve causes mitral insufficiency with regurgitation, which is often called mitral regurgitation (Fig. 4).

Repeated blood regurgitation in each cardiac cycle creates chronic pressure and volume overload of the atrium, eventually causing atrial dilation. In an effort to sustain arterial circulatory volume, the left ventricle must pump more blood to compensate for the regurgitant volume that flows backwards into the left atrium (Fig. 5).

Because this is a progressive degenerative disease, the volume of regurgitated blood increases over time, and the heart mounts increasing efforts to compensate, which eventually results in congestive heart failure (CHF).

Figure 5

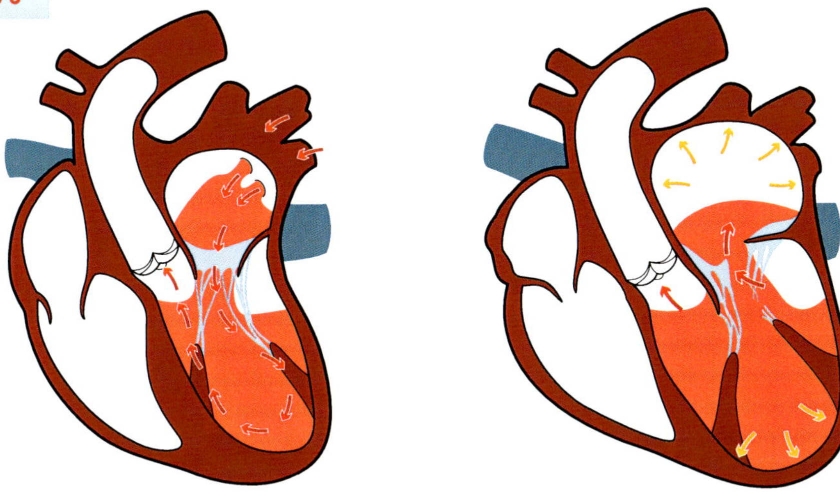

Mitral valve insufficiency allows blood regurgitation into the left atrium, resulting in its dilation. The increased volume of blood entering the ventricle to compensate for this situation also results in anatomical changes to the left ventricle.

Although this guide focuses only on CVD, atrioventricular regurgitation can result from alterations of the valve components cause by other pathologies, such as:

- Dilation of the valvular annulus due to ventricular dilation secondary to dilated cardiomyopathy.
- Anomalies of the atrioventricular valve leaflets due to congenital heart defects or bacterial endocarditis.
- Alterations of the chordae tendineae such as thinning, distension, or rupture.
- Damage to the papillary muscles secondary to hypertrophic cardiomyopathy.

Mitral valve degeneration alone	68 %
Mitral and tricuspid valve degeneration	8.5 %
Mitral and aortic valve degeneration	2.5 %
Tricuspid valve degeneration alone	1.3 %
Aortic valve degeneration alone	1.3 %

Table 1. Distribution of chronic valvular degeneration (Buchanan, J).

Although the mitral valve is typically affected, these pathological changes can also affect other valves (Table 1). Lesions of these other valves are similar to those of the mitral valve, though they tend to be less severe.

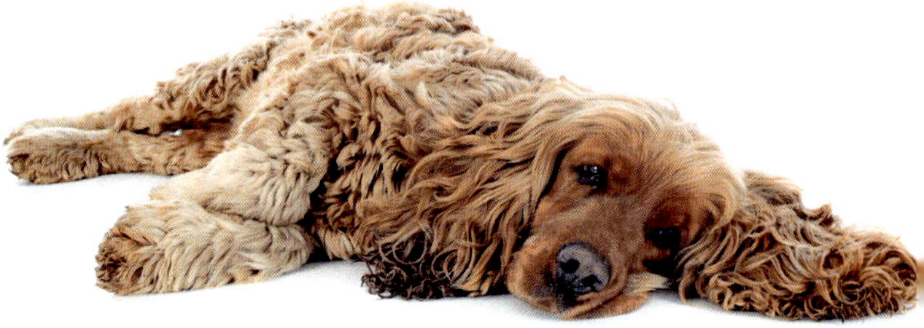

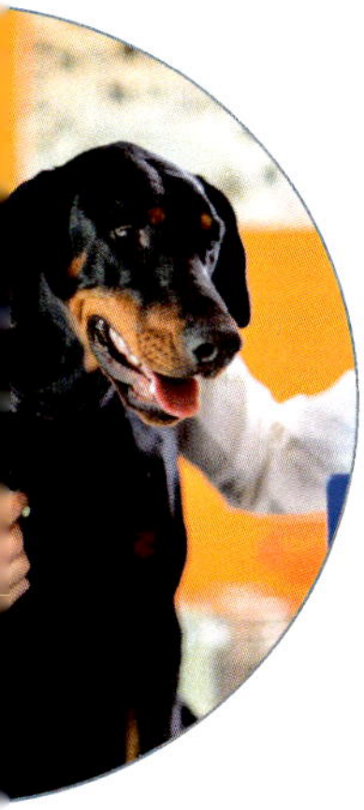

WHAT IS
CONGESTIVE HEART FAILURE?

Congestive heart failure (CHF) is the most common form of heart failure in dogs.

Many heart diseases, both acquired and congenital, can produce CHF, but the most common in dogs is CVD.

In this degenerative disease, chronic pressure and volume overload activates compensatory mechanisms in an effort to sustain cardiac function within normal limits. Over time, these mechanisms fail and trigger CHF, which eventually causes remodelling of the cardiac chambers.

Since surgical correction or transplantation of the diseased valve is not an option in CVD, the clinician's goal is to combat CHF, initially by delaying the subclinical, asymptomatic period and later by minimising and mitigating the deleterious effects of CVD that contribute to CHF.

DEFINITION

Congestive heart failure is a clinical condition in which the heart is unable to perform its functions; this generates venous congestion, which is the main cause of the observed clinical signs.

Pathophysiologically, the specific aetiology of the eventual heart disease is irrelevant. Whether it is due to a congenital abnormal communication, insufficient valve closure due to a degenerative process, or a disease of the myocardium, the consequences are the same: the heart initiates compensatory mechanisms to sustain cardiac output.

In other words, in patients with CVD and heart disease in general, except in rare cases, we treat not the specific lesion causing the heart disease, but rather its chronic pathophysiological consequences including CHF.

Depending on the type of heart disease, which side of the heart is affected, and whether systolic or diastolic function is more compromised, treatment protocols may vary, but CHF treatment generally involves the same components.

In CVD, which affects the left side of the heart, CHF results from an increase in pulmonary venous and left atrial pressures, leading to pulmonary oedema. The treatment should focus on managing these clinical signs.

PATHOPHYSIOLOGY
OF CONGESTIVE HEART FAILURE

1. As described, blood regurgitation from the left ventricle to the left atrium leads to chronic pressure and volume overload in the left cardiac chambers and a decrease in cardiac output equal to the regurgitated volume.
2. The body immediately discerns these changes and launches defensive systems in an effort to sustain cardiac output and blood pressure. These compensatory mechanisms can control the situation, but only in early stages and for brief durations.
3. Because the cause of the heart disease is not eliminated – rather, it persists or worsens over time – these systems ultimately lead to undesirable consequences more often than improvements in the haemodynamic status of CVD patients.

4. The cardiac dysfunction described results in hypoperfusion that does not satisfy the animal's metabolic needs. This triggers compensatory physiological mechanisms from the following two systems:
   - Sympathetic nervous system (SNS).
   - Renin–angiotensin–aldosterone system (RAAS).
5. This neuroendocrine response is initially effective but ultimately leads to clinical signs of CHF due to venous congestion. Congestive signs (cough, dyspnoea) arise from pulmonary oedema and, in advanced cases, signs of low cardiac output (weakness, syncope) occur.

CONSEQUENCES
OF THE COMPENSATORY MECHANISMS

The consequences of CHF compensatory mechanisms, which are under neuroendocrine regulation, are summarised below (Fig. 6).

Increase in sympathetic tone

This mechanism begins almost immediately and is the same one that is triggered when tissue oxygen demand increases for physiological (exercise, stress) or pathological (haemorrhage, hypovolaemia) reasons. Its purpose is to respond to brief, reversible emergency situations.

- Increase in heart rate (HR): the heart pumps more times per minute to compensate for the blood volume regurgitated into the left atrium so that normal cardiac output (CO) is maintained.
- Vasoconstriction (VC): increase in peripheral venous resistance to maintain systemic blood pressure. In this way, adequate perfusion of essential organs can be maintained with a decreased systolic volume, at the cost of increasing the work required for emptying the left ventricle – in other words, by increasing the preload.

Figure 6 CONGESTIVE HEART FAILURE PATHOPHYSIOLOGY

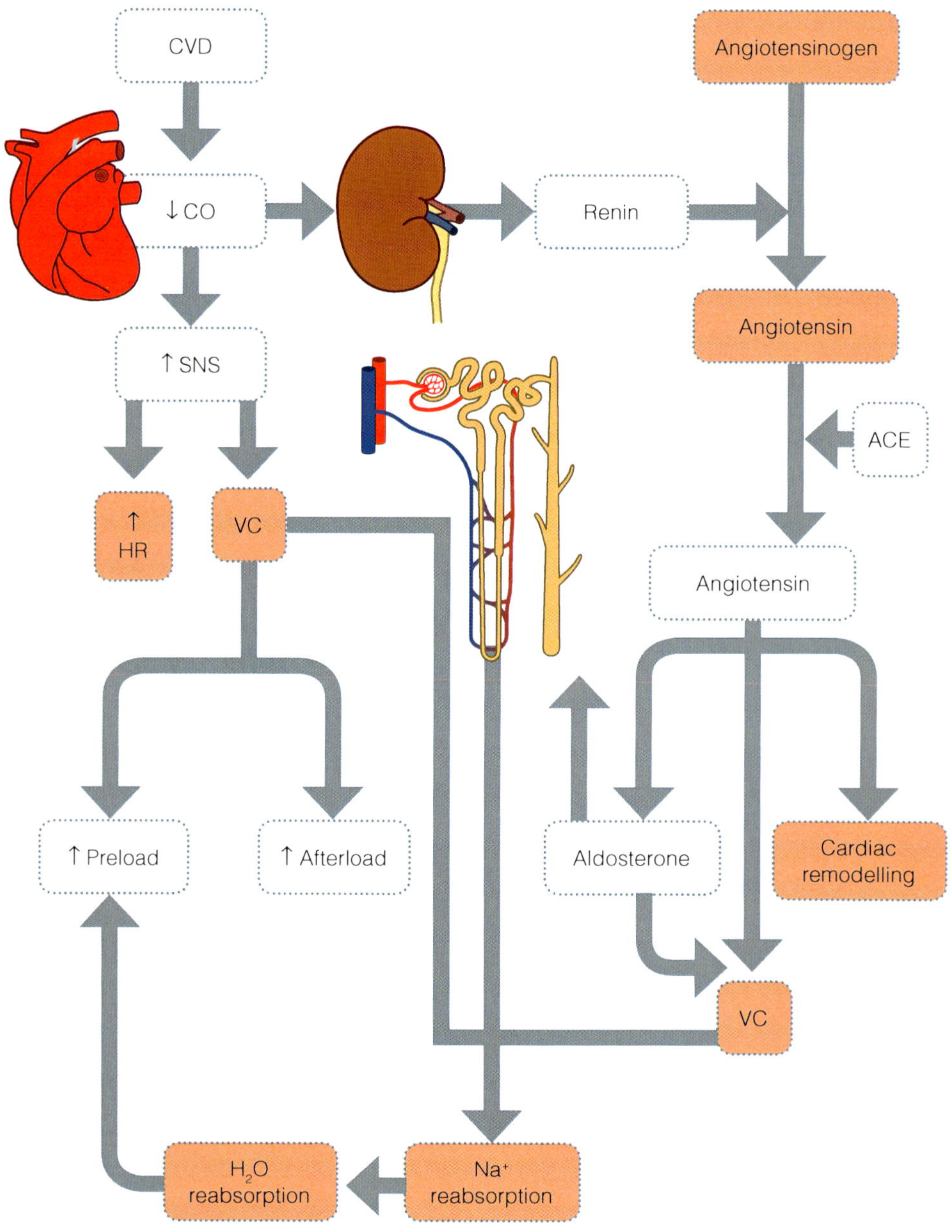

CVD, chronic valvular disease; CO, cardiac output; SNS, sympathetic nervous system; HR, heart rate; VC, vasoconstriction; ACE, angiotensin-converting enzyme.

RAAS activation

This is initiated later and is more effective and sustainable over time. The process is as follows:

- Angiotensinogen, which is inactive, is produced in the liver and released into the bloodstream.
- When mitral reflux decreases cardiac output or blood pressure, the baroreceptors of the renal juxtaglomerular apparatus release renin.
- Renin cleaves angiotensinogen to form angiotensin I, which is converted into angiotensin II by angiotensin-converting enzyme (ACE) in the lungs.
- Angiotensin II is an active hormone with several functions:
  - It is a powerful direct vasoconstrictor and SNS stimulant, which further increases the selective vasoconstriction of peripheral arterioles and veins.
  - It plays a role in the alteration of the vascular endothelium, fibrosis, and vascular and myocardial remodelling.
  - It stimulates aldosterone secretion by the adrenal glands. The release of aldosterone causes renal sodium retention and the release of anti-diuretic hormone (ADH) to enhance renal water retention, which in turn temporarily maintains cardiac output and enhances adrenergic tone.

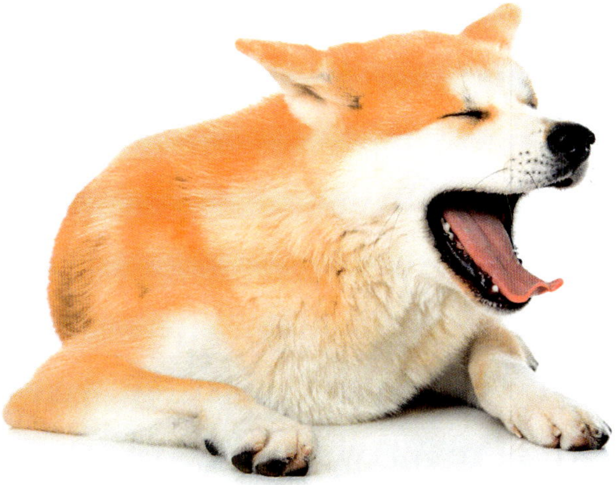

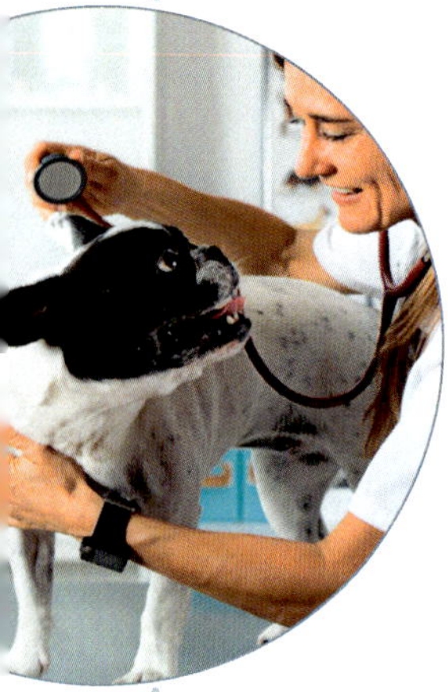

SUMMARY

The decrease in cardiac output due to mitral regurgitation and mitral insufficiency triggers the compensatory mechanisms that increase preload and afterload in order to maintain cardiac function.

Following a subclinical period that can last several years, the progression of valvular disease causes these measures to fail and triggers a vicious cycle (Fig. 7).

As cardiac function deteriorates, the neuroendocrine response increases, and as the neuroendocrine response increases, cardiac function further deteriorates:

- Increased preload involves greater systolic effort, which leads to left ventricular hypertrophy and dilation over time.
- The increase in preload, that is, in the circulating volume that a dilated left atrium must mobilise, leads to pulmonary oedema from congestion of the pulmonary vessels. If the tricuspid valve is also affected, generalised venous congestion may result, causing ascites, hepatomegaly, pleural effusion, or peripheral effusions.

Figure 7 VICIOUS CYCLE OF CONGESTIVE HEART FAILURE

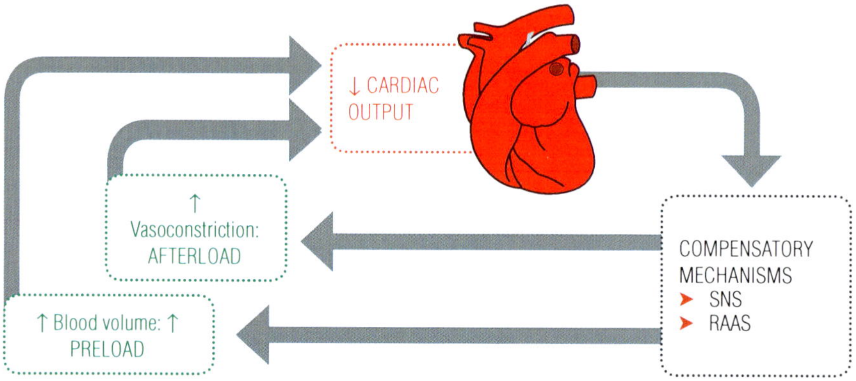

SNS, sympathetic nervous system; RAAS, renin–angiotensin–aldosterone system.

CLINICAL SIGNS OF CHRONIC VALVULAR DISEASE

For the reasons discussed, left-sided congestive signs (related to pulmonary oedema) predominate in CVD due to left-sided diastolic failure.

Signs of systolic failure can occur in dogs with very advanced CVD, but these appear late and in conjunction with the classic signs of cough and dyspnoea from pulmonary oedema. These signs of low cardiac output are the result of insufficient tissue oxygen delivery, with the resulting signs dependent on the organ affected:

- In the kidney, prerenal insufficiency occurs, with oliguria, proteinuria, azotaemia, and water and sodium retention due to hypoxic glomerular injury.
- In the central nervous system, dizziness, depression, drowsiness, and, in extreme cases, syncope, can occur; these may also be related to tachyarrhythmias.
- Hypoxia causes muscle weakness and asthaenia, which worsen exercise intolerance and fatigue and can lead to cardiac cachexia.
- Though uncommon, digestive signs such as nausea, vomiting, anorexia, diarrhoea-constipation, and maldigestion/malabsorption syndromes may occur at late stages, as well as increased liver enzymes due to hepatic congestion.

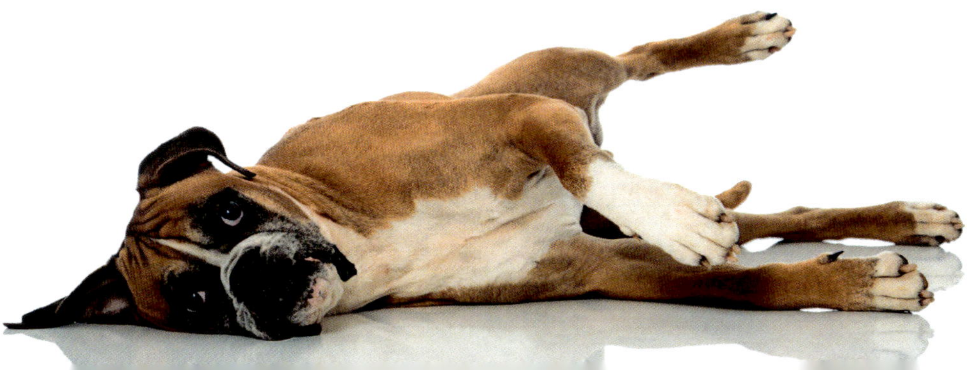

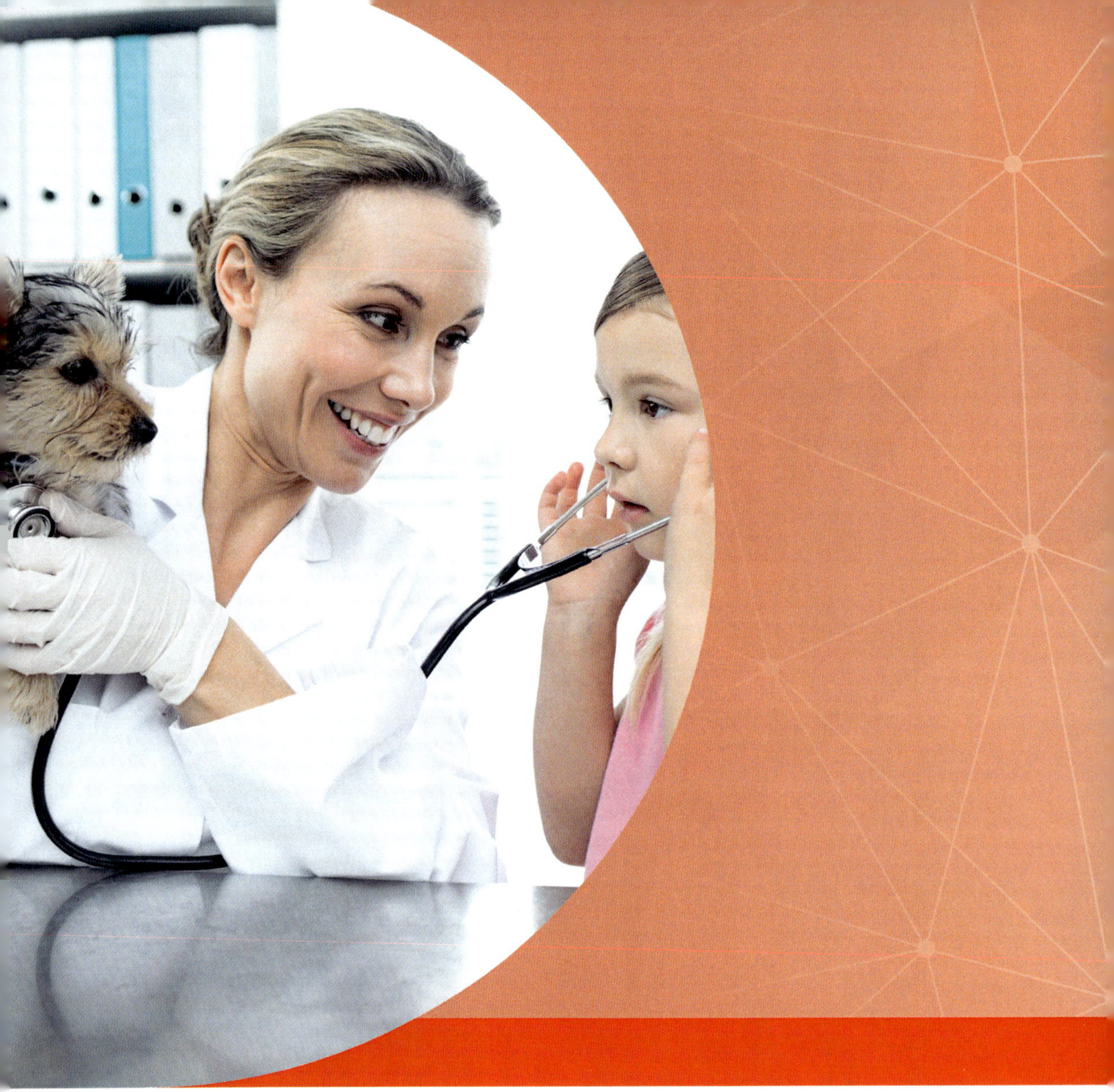

2

AT THE CLINIC

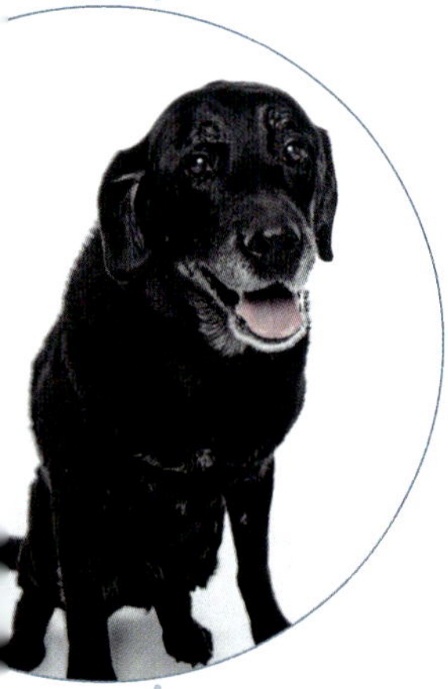

PREVALENCE
AND RISK FACTORS
OF CHRONIC VALVULAR DISEASE

Chronic valvular disease is extremely common in dogs and particularly affects elderly small-breed dogs.

> Approximately 10 % of all dogs present with some type of cardiac disease. Of these 10 %, 75 % are estimated to have CVD.

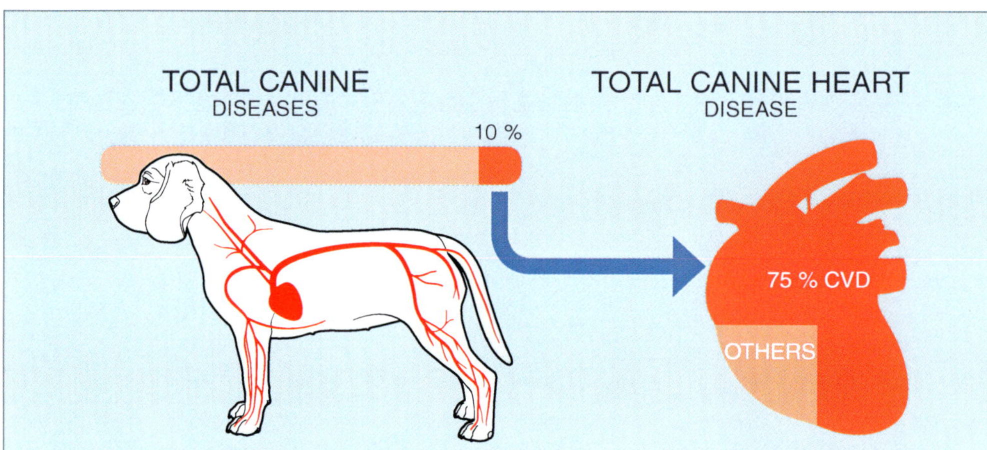

SIZE

The prevalence is much higher in miniature and small breeds, but it can affect dogs of any size.

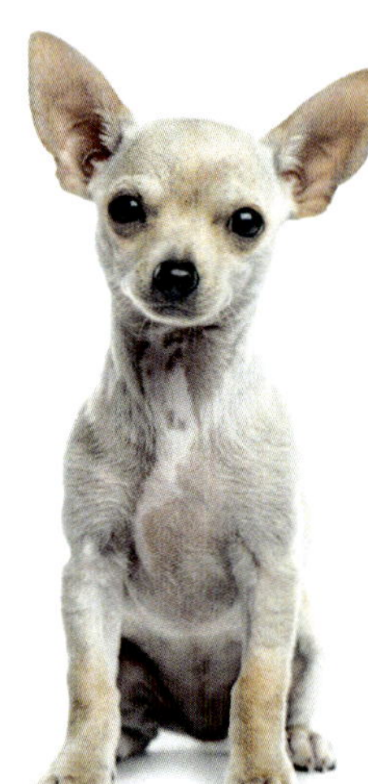

AGE

The prevalence of CVD rises significantly with age. In dogs 5–8 years of age it is approximately 10 %, rising to 20–25 % in dogs 9–12 years of age, and reaching 30–35 % in dogs older than 13. One recent study showed that 75 % of dogs older than 16 were affected.

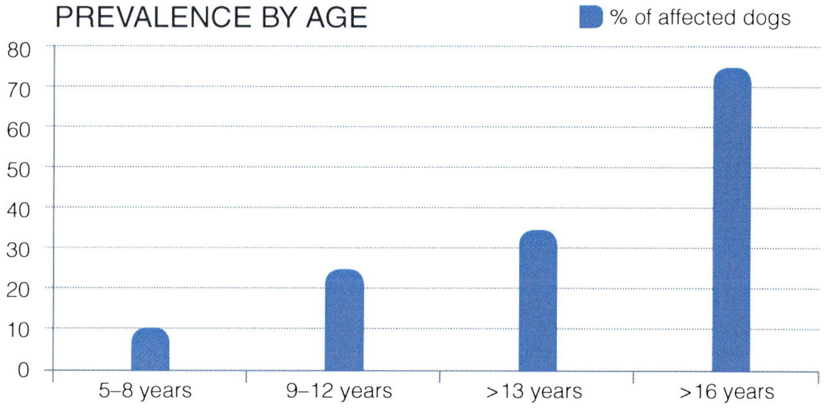

Chronic valvular disease is uncommon in patients under 5 years old. The disease is normally found by auscultation of a murmur in a dog 8–9 years old, but in certain breeds such as the Cavalier King Charles Spaniel or Norfolk Terrier, CVD can appear earlier, at a mean age of 6.25 years.

BREED

Chronic valvular disease can affect dogs of any breed, but studies have demonstrated a higher prevalence in certain ones.

Cavalier King Charles Spaniels are especially predisposed to CVD, and it can begin at a very young age in this breed; one study reported a prevalence of 10 % in patients under one year old, 56 % in dogs under age five, and 100 % in those aged 10 and over.

HIGHEST BREED PREDISPOSITIONS	
Cavalier King Charles Spaniel	Fox Terrier
Poodle	Pekingese
Dachshund	Boston Terrier
Chihuahua	Norfolk Terrier
Pomeranian	Miniature Schnauzer
Yorkshire Terrier	Cocker Spaniel
Lhasa Apso	Dobermann Pinscher
Shi-tzu	Small mixed-breed

CVD PREVALENCE BY AGE IN THE CAVALIER KING CHARLES SPANIEL

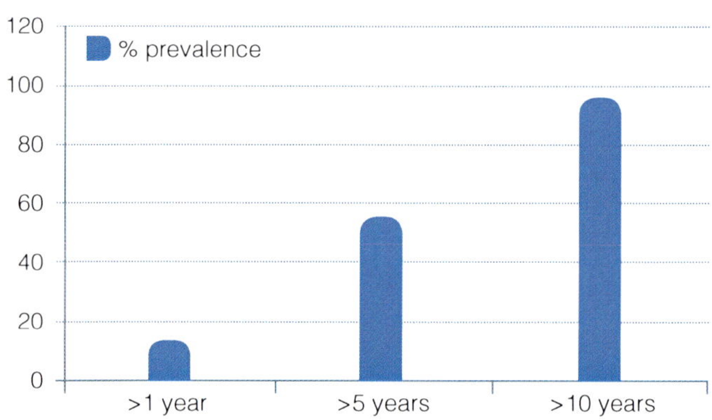

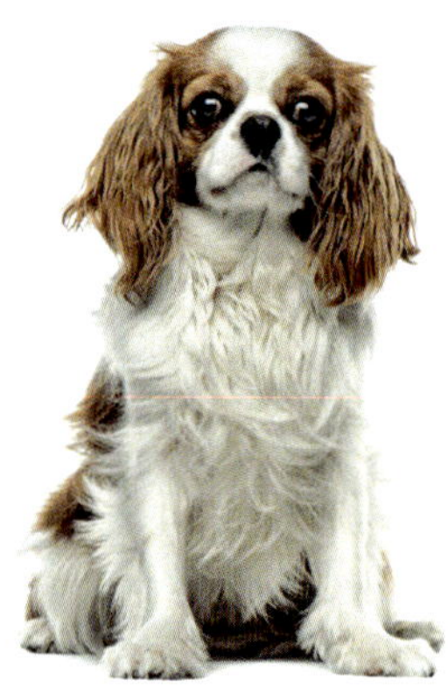

Chronic valvular disease is such a severe problem in Cavalier King Charles Spaniels that some breed clubs have started control programmes to prevent breeding of individuals with mitral regurgitation murmurs. Such programmes have proven effective for limiting the incidence of the disease.

SEX

Males are more prone to CVD than females, with a ratio of 1.5:1 in one study. Males tend to develop CVD at a younger age as well.

CLINICAL SIGNS

Chronic valvular disease is a chronic degenerative disease that worsens over time (Table 1).

CHRONIC VALVULAR DISEASE STAGES	
Early stage	**Late stage**
➤ A small volume of blood is regurgitated into the left atrium. ➤ The patient is able to compensate. ➤ No obvious clinical signs exist. ➤ May last several years.	➤ As the valve degenerates, the regurgitated volume increases. ➤ The neuroendocrine response induces fluid retention and congestion. ➤ Clinical signs appear. ➤ May last several years, and clinical signs tend to worsen over time.

Table 1. Chronic valvular disease stages

Most clinical signs attributed to CVD-related mitral regurgitation are due to pulmonary congestion. Patients with CVD and pulmonary congestion often present with marked respiratory distress. Cough is quite common but nonspecific for congestive heart failure (CHF) in dogs; it also occurs in respiratory diseases (chronic bronchitis, pulmonary fibrosis, tracheal collapse, bronchopneumonia, upper respiratory infections, etc.).

Exercise intolerance, cough, and dyspnoea are the most common presenting complaints in patients with CVD, though these are not the only ones. The table below shows the clinical signs that owners most often report (Table 2).

➤ Weakness, fatigue, apathy	➤ Inappetence, weight loss
➤ Difficulty breathing	➤ Syncope, weakness, pallor
➤ Cough	➤ Distended abdomen
➤ Nocturnal restlessness	

Table 2. Clinical signs owners most often describe.

None of these clinical signs is specific to CHF.

- Exercise intolerance, apathy, weakness, and anorexia are vague signs. In an elderly dog, they can signify multiple problems: degenerative, autoimmune, metabolic, endocrine, neoplastic, infectious, inflammatory, or traumatic lesions in any organ or system. They are not helpful in a differential diagnosis.
- An atypical breathing pattern may limit the problem to a respiratory or cardiac aetiology, but keep in mind other possible causes of abnormal breathing, such as acid-base imbalance, severe anaemia, or intense pain such as that of a herniated disc.
- Cough is the most informative clinical sign in CVD diagnosis in that it ensures a cardiac or respiratory aetiology. A cardiac cough is traditionally described as dry and occurring at night, but this is not always the case, nor is such a cough always due to cardiac disease. Coughs in CVD have two causes:
  - Compression of the left main bronchus by a dilated left atrium.
  - Pulmonary oedema.
- Syncope is not as common in CVD as in other cardiac diseases (subaortic stenosis, dilated cardiomyopathy, etc.), and it tends to occur only in very advanced disease as a result of arrhythmias or decompensation due to ruptured chordae tendinae of the leaflets.
- Ascites and other peripheral effusions may be signs of right-sided CHF or other noncardiac pathologies (neoplasms, liver failure, kidney disease, etc.). These are uncommon in CVD, since it is usually the left atrioventricular (mitral) valve that is affected. Tricuspid valve disease rarely occurs in isolation; if present it is usually seen with long-standing advanced mitral valve disease.

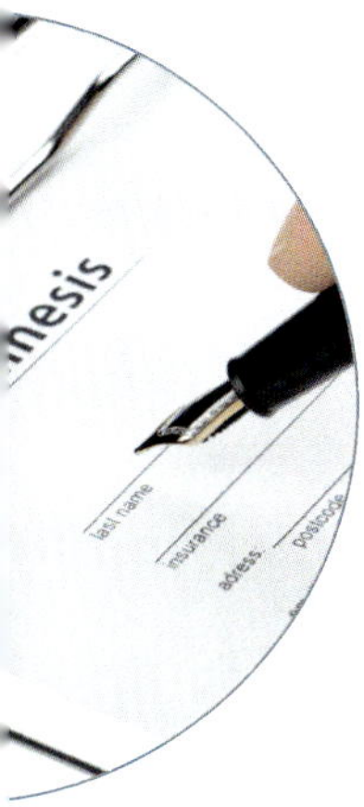

HISTORY

Once the clinical signs are identified, the history (Fig. 1) should narrow down the differential diagnoses:

- Describe the clinical signs in detail. How long have they been present, when did they start, duration, severity, progression, etc.
- Are they correlated to any factor? Exercise, rest, stress, feeding, time of year, etc.
- Are there other clinical signs atypical of CHF that may indicate a non-cardiac disease? Vomiting, diarrhoea, seizures, lameness, fever, polydipsia, polyuria.
- Has a parent or littermate had cardiac disease?
- Vaccination and antiparasite history?
- Has the patient been in contact with other dogs or stayed in an area where a particular infectious or parasitic disease such as heartworm is endemic?
- Have murmurs or arrhythmias been previously ausculted?
- Has the patient been given any medication? If so, what was the response?
- Is there any recent or previous history of trauma or possible toxicity?
- Is there any previously diagnosed chronic disease? Tumours, metabolic or endocrine diseases, etc.

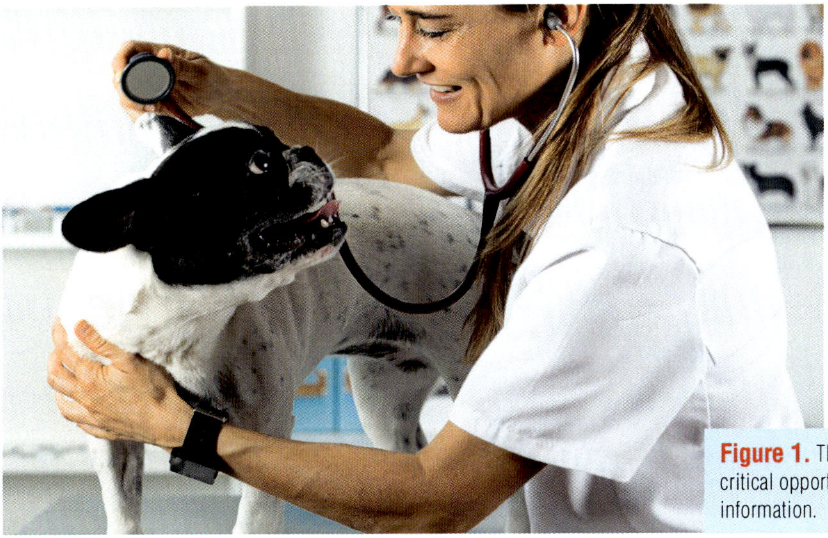

Figure 1. The history is a critical opportunity for collecting information.

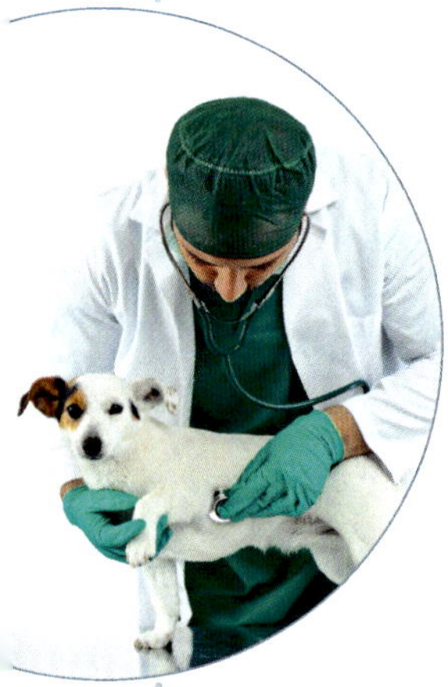

PHYSICAL EXAMINATION

GENERAL CLINICAL EXAMINATION

Maintain a consistent approach, even if the information in the history clearly hints of a potential cardiopulmonary aetiology. A nonsystematic approach may overlook clinical findings relevant to less likely diagnoses, as well as the presence of comorbidities.

CARDIOVASCULAR EXAMINATION

After the general examination, a cardiovascular examination is performed that is more extensive than that of a routine consultation. The cardiovascular examination includes three steps:

1. General examination

- Body condition: dogs with advanced CHF due to CVD may lose weight, but cachexia is not as common as in other heart diseases such as dilated cardiomyopathy. Obesity is a risk factor for cough in dogs with cardiac and respiratory disease.
- Palpable lymph nodes and masses that can indicate neoplasms or metastases.
- Possible free abdominal fluid, although CVD generally causes left-sided CHF, which does not give rise to ascites.
- Mucous membrane colour (conjunctival and oral):
  - Pale mucous membranes may result from vasoconstriction and low cardiac output, indicating cardiac decompensation.
  - Injected mucous membranes may result from right-sided CHF (less common with CVD).
  - Cyanotic mucous membranes can occur due to severe respiratory disease (for example, airway obstruction) or severe congenital heart disease.

- Slow capillary refill time suggests decreased cardiac output.
- Ocular and nasal discharge suggests infectious respiratory disease.
- Jugular distension and jugular pulse are associated with right-sided CHF. Heartworm, congenital right heart disease, right atrial haemangiosarcoma, and pericardial effusion rarely occur with CVD.
- Tracheal palpation and whether it causes the animal to cough.

2. Breathing pattern and resting respiratory rate

The breathing pattern and respiratory rate are very important not only to differentiate between respiratory and cardiac disease, but also to determine disease severity and monitor dogs with a prior diagnosis of CVD-induced CHF (Table 3).

Resting breathing pattern

TIPS FOR EVALUATING BREATHING PATTERNS
➤ Do not confuse with physiological panting, which is a normal result of increased body heat, exercise, and stress of the examination.
➤ Inspiratory dyspnoea often signifies upper airway obstruction.
➤ Expiratory dyspnoea may indicate tracheal collapse, intrathoracic masses, or severe pulmonary oedema.
➤ Dyspnoea due to cardiogenic pulmonary oedema may be inspiratory, upon exertion, or expiratory, so it cannot be distinguished from dyspnoea due to other lung diseases such as bronchopneumonia.
➤ Orthopnoea is characterised by a posture in which the dog refuses to lie down and remains standing or seated, neck extended, nose turned upwards, and elbows separated (Fig. 2). Its most common cause is acute pulmonary oedema from decompensated CVD-induced CHF; it is always a medical emergency.

Table 3. Breathing pattern assessment.

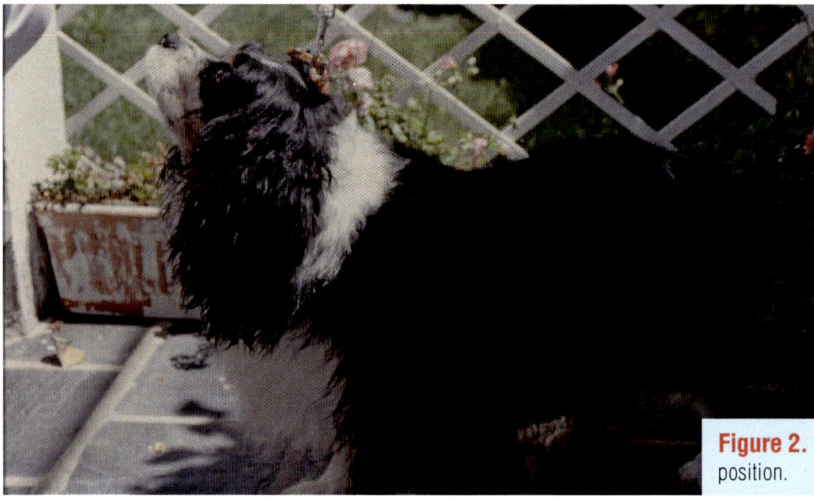

Figure 2. Dog in orthopnoeic position.

A respiratory rate measured in the clinic is understandably not very accurate due to the animal's stress. In contrast, a rate taken by an owner at home is more useful.

Resting respiratory rate

The resting respiratory rate (RRR) is the number of breaths per minute in an awake, calm patient; alternatively, a sleeping respiratory rate (SRR) can be measured (Tables 4 and 5). These are useful, valuable tools.

Monitoring RRR and SRR at home is generally the best way for owners to detect cardiac decompensation early.

The objective of monitoring the patient's resting respiratory rate is to detect any worsening of the disease before the next follow-up visit and to prevent hospitalisations and deaths from CHF (Graph 1).

Studies have shown a correlation between increased RRR and SRR and having CHF, and these measurements are comparable in efficacy to those of much more complex modalities such as echocardiography, cardiac biomarkers, and clinical examination.

	Normal reference range (bpm)	Mean normal reference values (bpm)
RRR	15–35	19
SRR	6–25	15

Table 4. Resting respiratory rate (RRS) and sleeping respiratory rate (SRR) reference values in healthy dogs, as measured by owners at home.

The lower limits are not diagnostically useful, but the upper limits are predictive of CHF.

A SRR above 25 bpm or a RRR above 35 bpm over several days is predictive of decompensated CHF and indicates a need for immediate medical care.

INSTRUCTIONS FOR OWNERS
➤ Owners should measure RRR or SRR, whichever is easier. Sleeping respiratory rate measurement is usually easier for most people.
➤ Teach owners how to count a full breathing cycle during the appointment, and refer owners to educational videos online. Count the number of breaths in 30 seconds and double it, with the dog resting while recumbent (RRR) or sleeping (SRR).
➤ The patient should be calm and not have exercised in the previous 30 minutes. The dog should have been asleep for at least 15 minutes prior to measuring SRR. If the dog is panting, the count is invalid.
➤ Measure RRR or SRR daily or at least twice per week, under the same conditions and at the same times, preferably by the same person.
➤ Record the data on a card or using an application for electronic devices.
➤ If the patient is stable, results from the first week may serve as a reference for future measurements.
➤ If two or three consecutive measurements exceed the reference value by 25 % or surpass the upper limit provided in Table 1, this may signal decompensated CHF, and the patient should be seen at the clinic.

Table 5. Instructions for owners of dogs with chronic valvular disease.

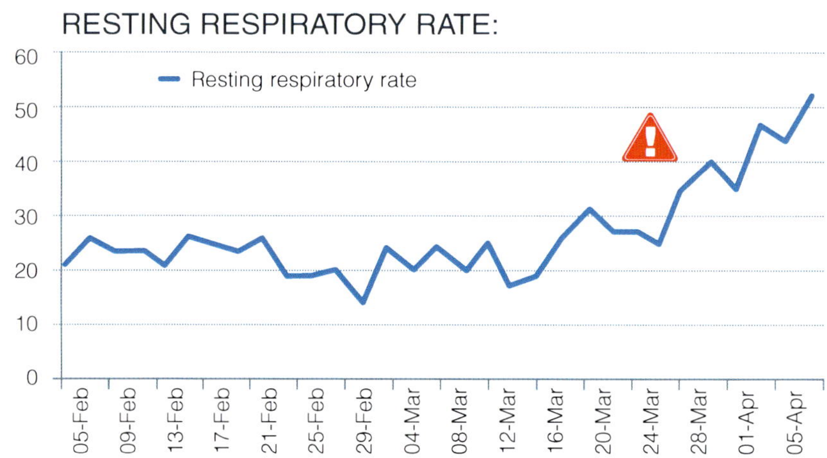

Graph 1. Monitoring the resting respiratory rate empowers owners to quickly detect decompensation when this rate exceeds 30–35 bpm, as in the case shown here.

3. Auscultation and cardiac pulse

Under normal conditions, blood flow through the heart is silent because the blood molecules move in parallel. This is known as laminar flow. In CVD, defective valve closure produces blood regurgitation from the left ventricle to the left atrium, causing turbulence (Fig. 3). This turbulent flow causes a regurgitation murmur during ventricular systole, the phase of the cardiac cycle when the atrioventricular valves should be completely closed to allow blood to exit the ventricles via the major arteries (Fig. 4). Mitral murmurs are always systolic; that is, they occur between S1 and S2 (Fig. 5).

Figure 3

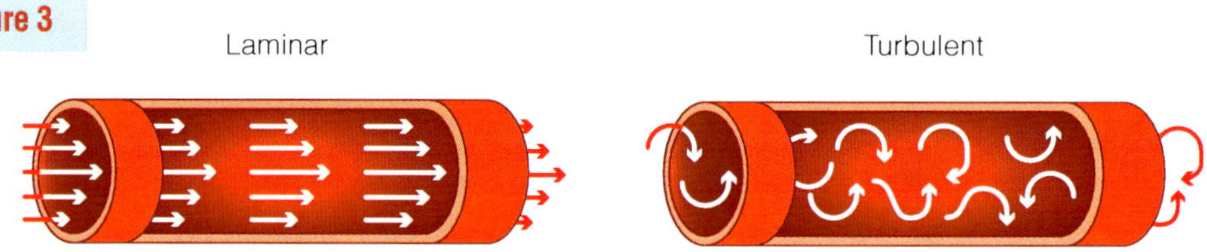

In chronic valvular disease, blood flow through the heart is turbulent.

Figure 4 MITRAL MURMUR

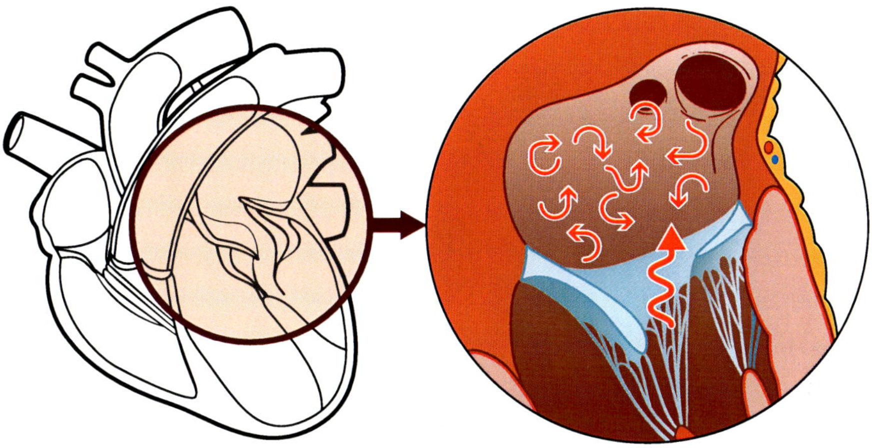

In chronic valvular disease, the atrioventricular valves do not close completely, producing a mitral murmur.

Figure 5 MITRAL MURMUR

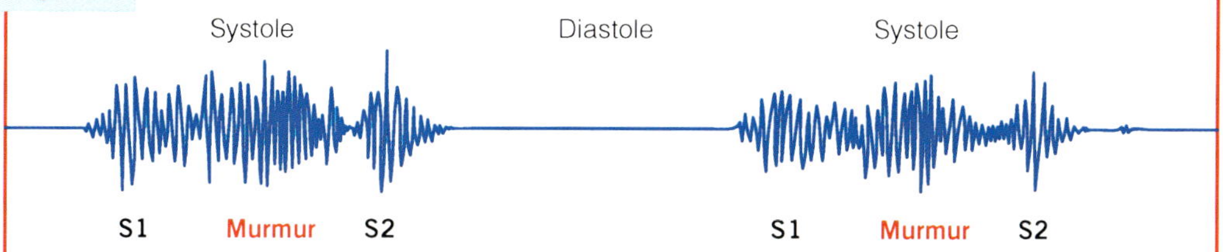

The mitral murmur that occurs in chronic valvular disease is systolic; it occurs between the first and second heart sounds (S1 and S2).

Cardiac auscultation is the most practical, economical, simple, and noninvasive technique to detect CVD as well as the key to early diagnosis of asymptomatic dogs.

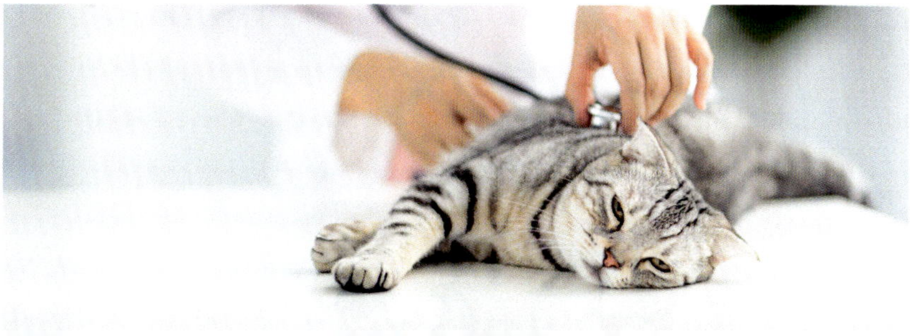

Auscultation allows detection of normal heart sounds, evaluation of the heart rate and rhythm, and identification of murmurs and other abnormalities.

AUSCULTATION CHARACTERISTICS IN A CVD PATIENT

- The first sign in dogs with early CVD is a mild, grade I/VI or II/VI holosystolic murmur with maximal intensity in the mitral area at the left fifth intercostal space (Table 6).
- In some moderate CVD cases, the murmur is intermittent and appears only at the end of inspiration. A systolic click may occur in mid-systole (mesosystolic click) or at the end of systole (telesystolic click). Sometimes it is the first anomaly detected on auscultation, before a systolic murmur appears.
- In Cavalier King Charles Spaniels, the intensity of the heart murmur, heart size, severity of regurgitation, and clinical stage of the disease are closely linked. In other breeds, the intensity of the murmur is a less reliable indicator of the extent of the valvular lesion.
- Mitral regurgitation murmurs are more intense during physical exercise and stress, and they can become quite soft or even disappear in advanced CHF.
- As the mitral regurgitation murmur becomes more intense, the sound tends to radiate dorsally, cranially, caudally and to the right.
  Therefore, it is particularly difficult to differentiate a tricuspid murmur from a murmur of mitral origin that has radiated to the right.
- Cardiac arrhythmias can alter the intensity of a murmur by interrupting the normal heart rhythm. Auscult or palpate the point of maximum impulse while taking the femoral pulse to detect pulse deficits suggestive of arrhythmias.
- The pulse of dogs with CVD may be powerful and brief.
- Respiratory sinus arrhythmia is physiological in the dog and quite pronounced in healthy dogs at rest, particularly in brachycephalic breeds with high vagal tone.
  Do not confuse it with pathological arrhythmias.
- Once cardiac compensation mechanisms initiate, the heart rate increases and sinus arrhythmia disappears, as discussed in Chapter 3.
- Patients with advanced CHF may have crepitations on auscultation due to pulmonary oedema, but these lung sounds are not unique to CHF and can result from respiratory diseases such as pulmonary hypertension, bronchitis, and bronchopneumonia.

Differential diagnosis of left-sided murmur	
Cause of murmur	**Characteristics of murmur**
Subaortic stenosis*	Loudest in the aortic area: dorsocranial to the point of maximum impulse, at the base of the heart
Pulmonary stenosis*	Loudest in the pulmonary valve area: cranial to the aortic valve area
Interatrial communication*	Loudest at the base of the heart
Interventricular communication*	Often loudest on the left side, but the point of maximum intensity is usually in the right hemithorax.
Patent ductus arteriosus*	Usually a continuous or machinery murmur
Mitral regurgitation	Loudest in the mitral area. The most common cause is CVD, but it can appear in other diseases such as congenital dysplasia*, ventricular dilation secondary to dilated cardiomyopathy, and bacterial endocarditis.

Table 6. Differential diagnoses of left-sided murmurs

*Congenital heart disease. This murmur is identified in puppies and juvenile animals, in contrast to that of CVD (caution in juvenile Cavalier King Charles Spaniels).

The most common, but not the only, cause of murmur in the dog is mitral regurgitation. Murmur can occur in any congenital heart disease, bacterial endocarditis, or secondarily in dilated cardiomyopathy; murmurs can also be innocent or arise from anaemia, hypertension, hypoproteinaemia, etc.

See the diagnostic algorithm for murmurs in dogs on pages 32 and 33 for more information on the differential diagnosis of murmurs.

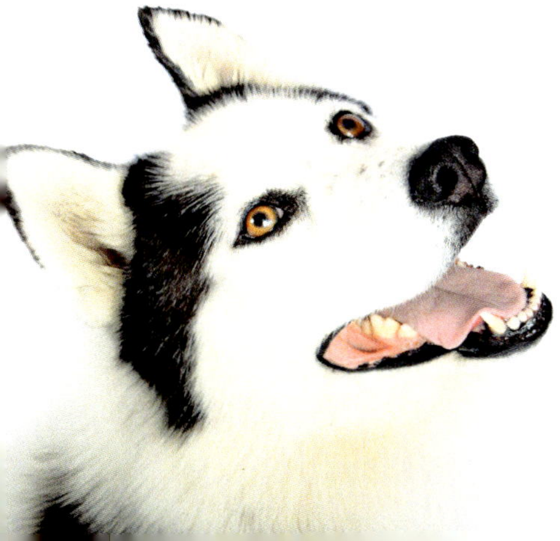

DIAGNOSTIC ALGORITHM OF MURMURS IN DOGS

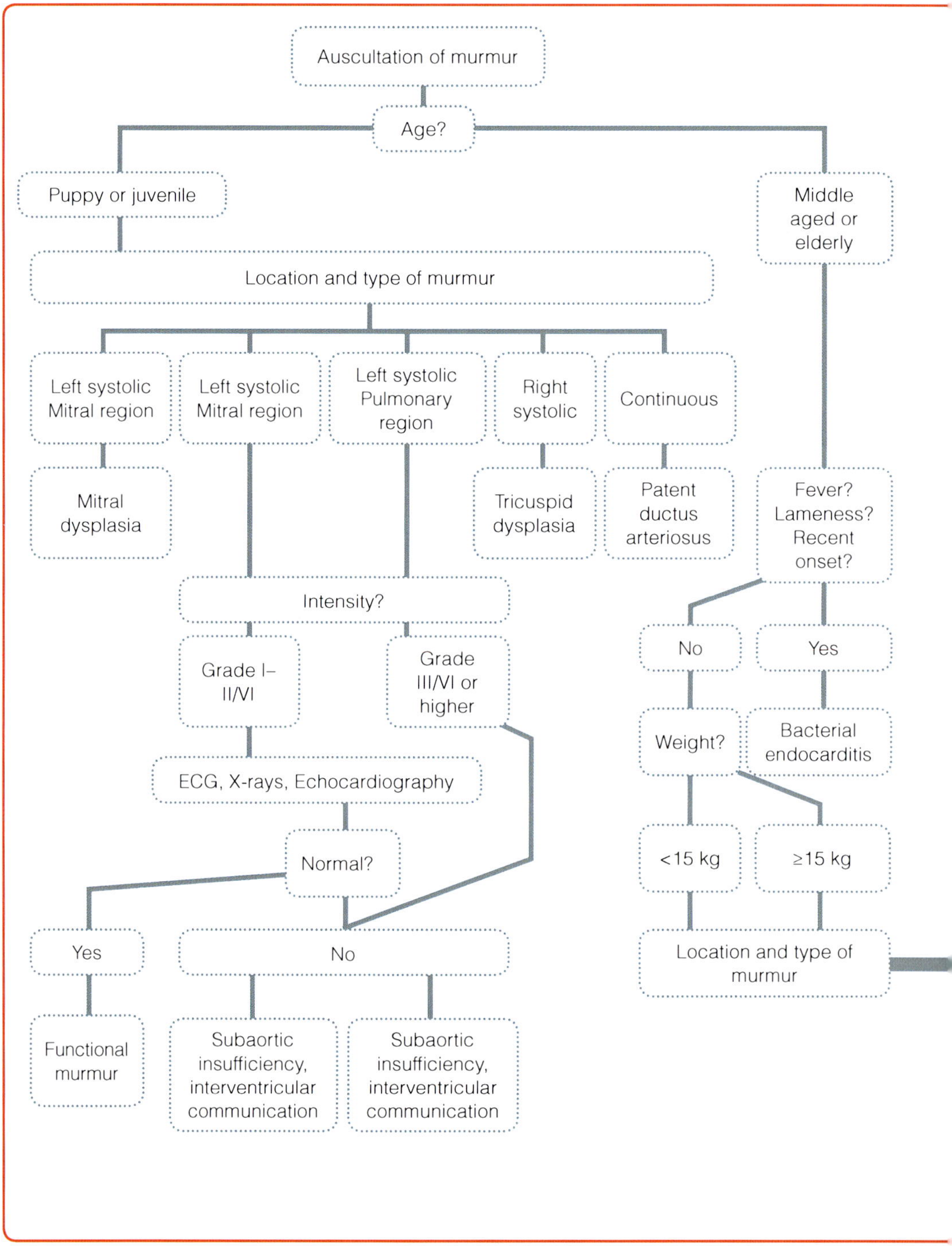

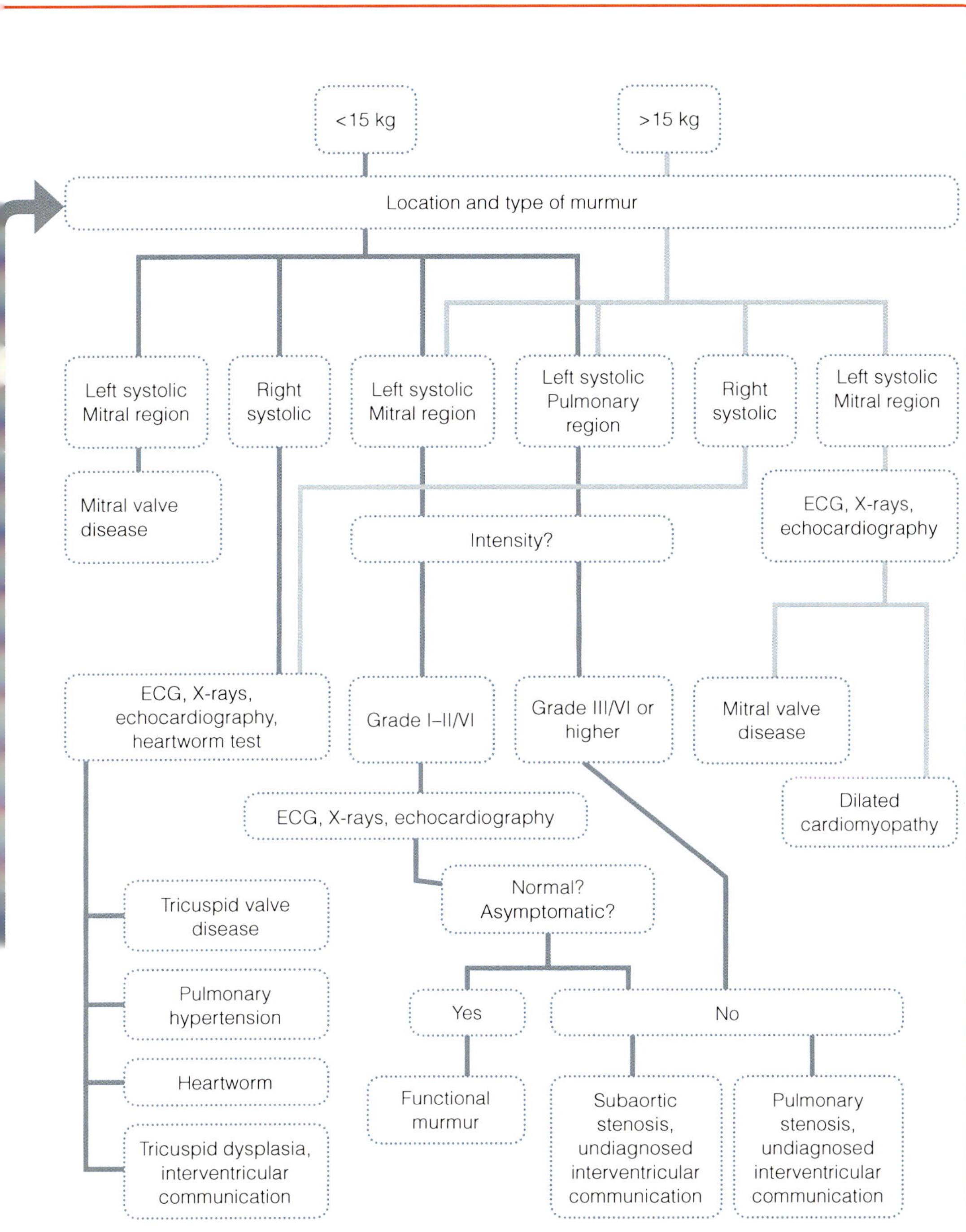
<15 kg
>15 kg
Location and type of murmur
Left systolic Mitral region
Right systolic
Left systolic Mitral region
Left systolic Pulmonary region
Right systolic
Left systolic Mitral region
Mitral valve disease
ECG, X-rays, echocardiography
Intensity?
ECG, X-rays, echocardiography, heartworm test
Grade I–II/VI
Grade III/VI or higher
Mitral valve disease
Dilated cardiomyopathy
ECG, X-rays, echocardiography
Normal? Asymptomatic?
Tricuspid valve disease
Pulmonary hypertension
Heartworm
Tricuspid dysplasia, interventricular communication
Yes
No
Functional murmur
Subaortic stenosis, undiagnosed interventricular communication
Pulmonary stenosis, undiagnosed interventricular communication

Auscultation step by step

Proper auscultation requires a standardised, systematic technique of sequential steps:

1. Choose a quiet environment without external noise to avoid stressing the patient. Sympathetic activation increases heart rate and contractility, potentially inducing turbulent flow. It also enhances movement and breathing artefacts.
2. During auscultation, heart sounds, breath sounds, and sounds from patient movement, rubbing of fur, background noise, etc., may occur. Clinicians must minimise interference from artefacts and maintain concentration to discriminate heart sounds.
3. Positioning: the patient should stand so the heart sits at its normal position, with the mouth open (Fig. 6).
4. Always follow the same order of auscultation of the anatomical heart regions. Use both the diaphragm and the bell of the stethoscope.
5. Two methods exist for localisation of auscultation zones:
   a. Various anatomical landmarks such as the shoulder or olecranon may be used for reference in standing patients. In this position, picture a horizontal line from the shoulder joint to just above the valve auscultation areas (Figs. 7 and 8).
   b. Palpation of the apex beat is a more accurate technique, as it does not depend on the forelimb position. The apex beat is the pulse felt at the point of maximum impulse at the beginning of the ventricular contraction, when the heart strikes the chest wall. It is palpated at the left fifth intercostal space and should be identified by palpation before starting the auscultation (Figs. 8 and 9).

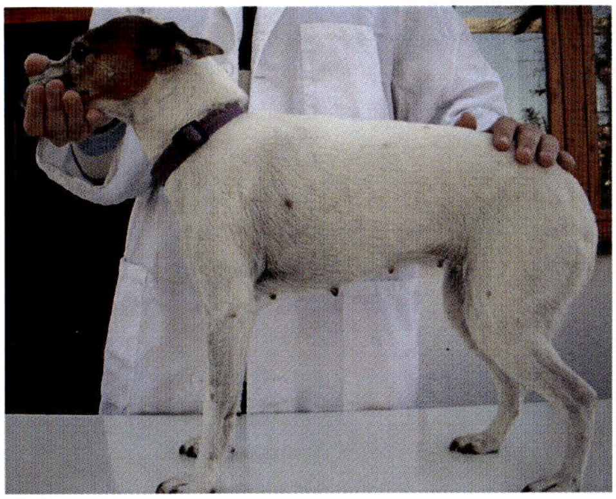

Figure 6. Example of proper body position for heart auscultation.

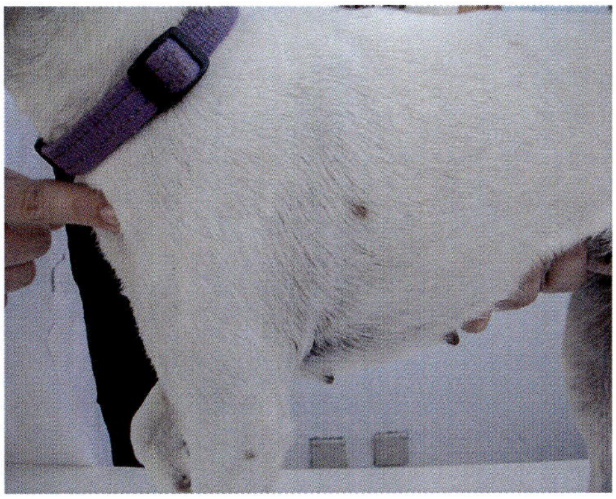

Figure 7. Imaginary horizontal line for localisation of auscultation regions.

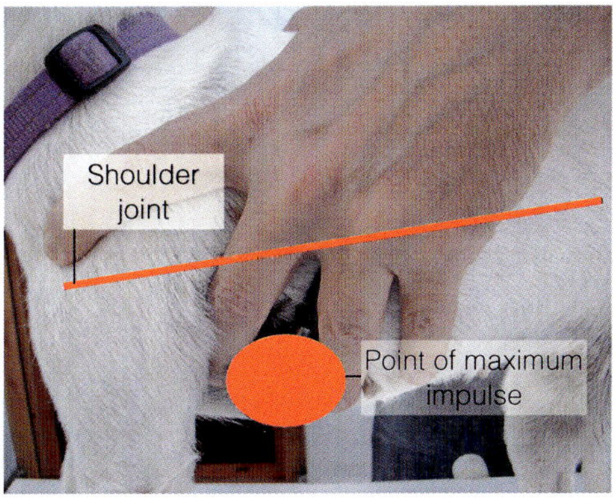

Figure 8. Two auscultation techniques are shown.

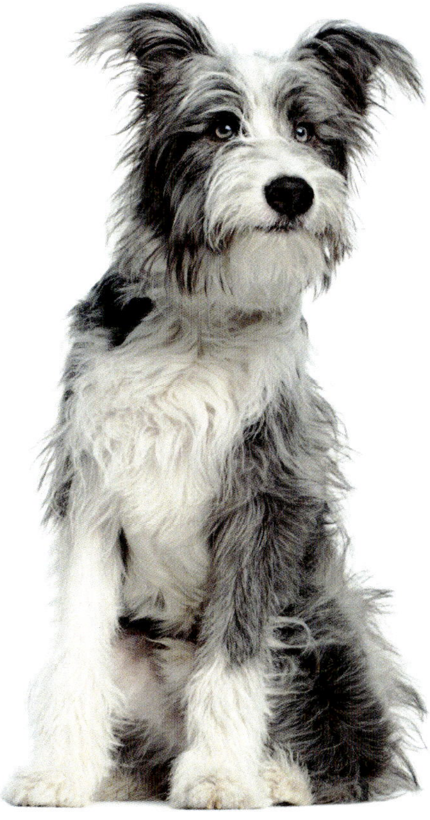

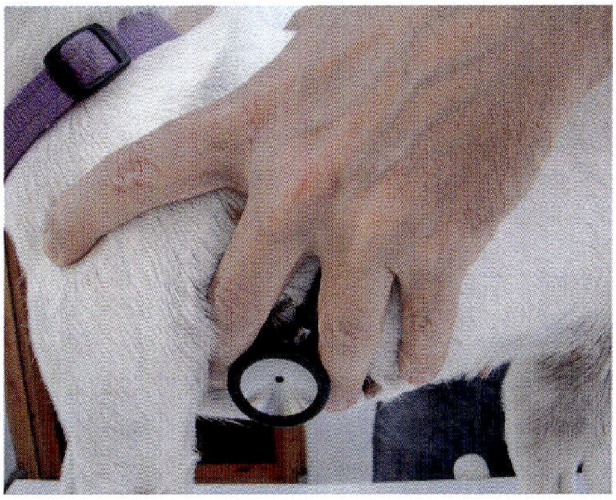

Figure 9. Palpation of the point of maximum impulse.

6. Auscult all areas of the heart: start on the left and use the acronym MAP as a guide (Fig. 10).
    - Mitral: left fifth intercostal space at the level of the costochondral junction. A mitral regurgitation murmur is loudest in the mitral area, but in late stages it can radiate to other areas including the right hemithorax, especially if the tricuspid valve is also affected (Fig. 11).
    - Aortic: left fourth intercostal space above the costochondral junction.
    - Pulmonary: left side between the second and fourth intercostal space just above the sternum.
    - Tricuspid: right side between the third and fifth intercostal space, near the costochondral junction (Fig. 12).
7. Locate the femoral pulse during cardiac auscultation. The pulse starts immediately after S1. One pulse should occur per heartbeat, and a pulse deficit is indicative of arrhythmia (premature ventricular or supraventricular complexes) due to incomplete ventricular filling (Fig. 13).

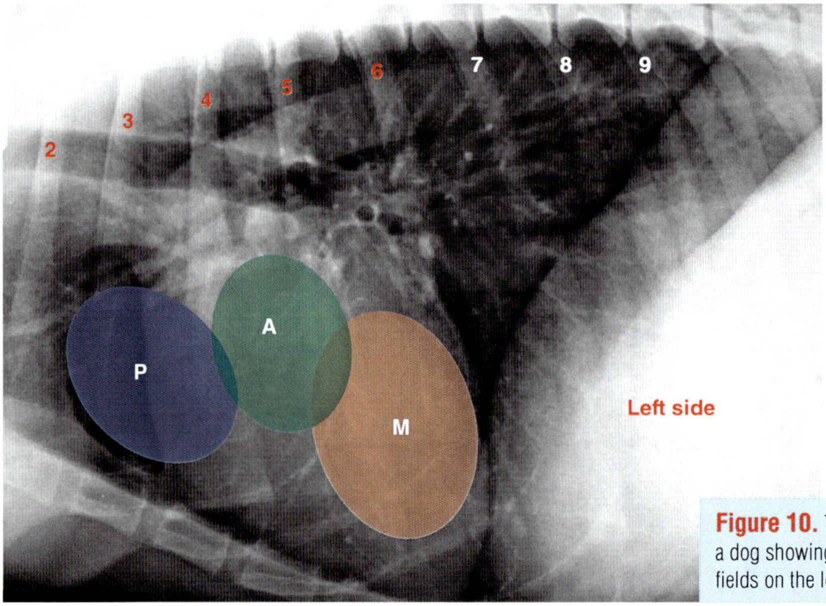

Figure 10. Thoracic X-ray of a dog showing all auscultation fields on the left side.

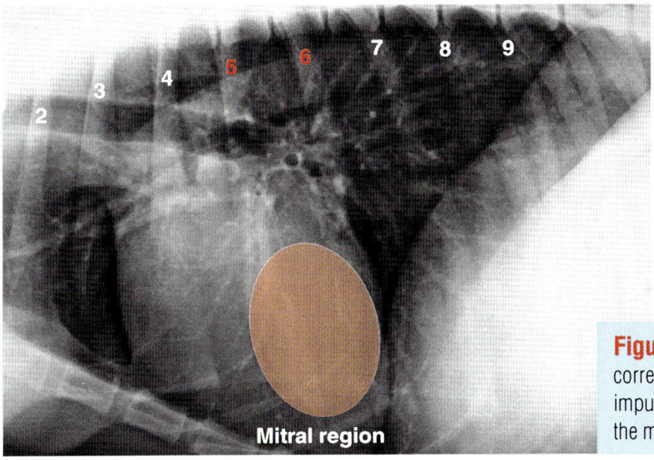

Figure 11. Mitral area in the left hemithorax, corresponding to the point of maximum impulse and the point of maximum intensity of the mitral regurgitation murmur.

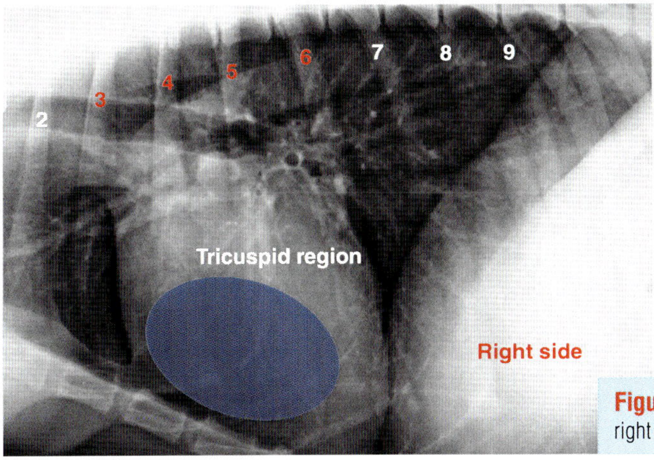

Figure 12. Tricuspid auscultation area in the right hemithorax.

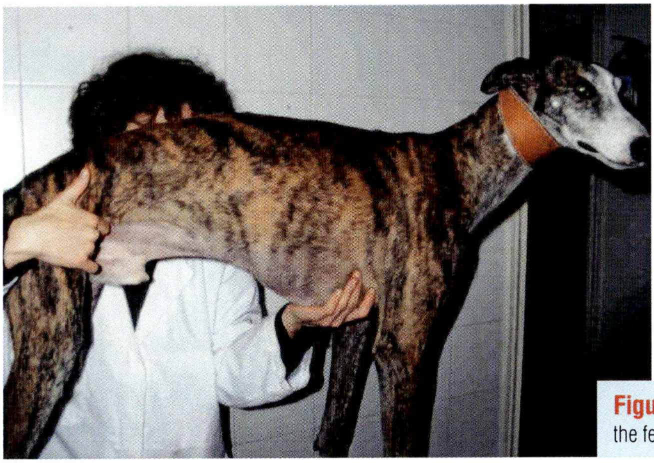

Figure 13. Illustration of how to measure the femoral and cardiac pulses simultaneously.

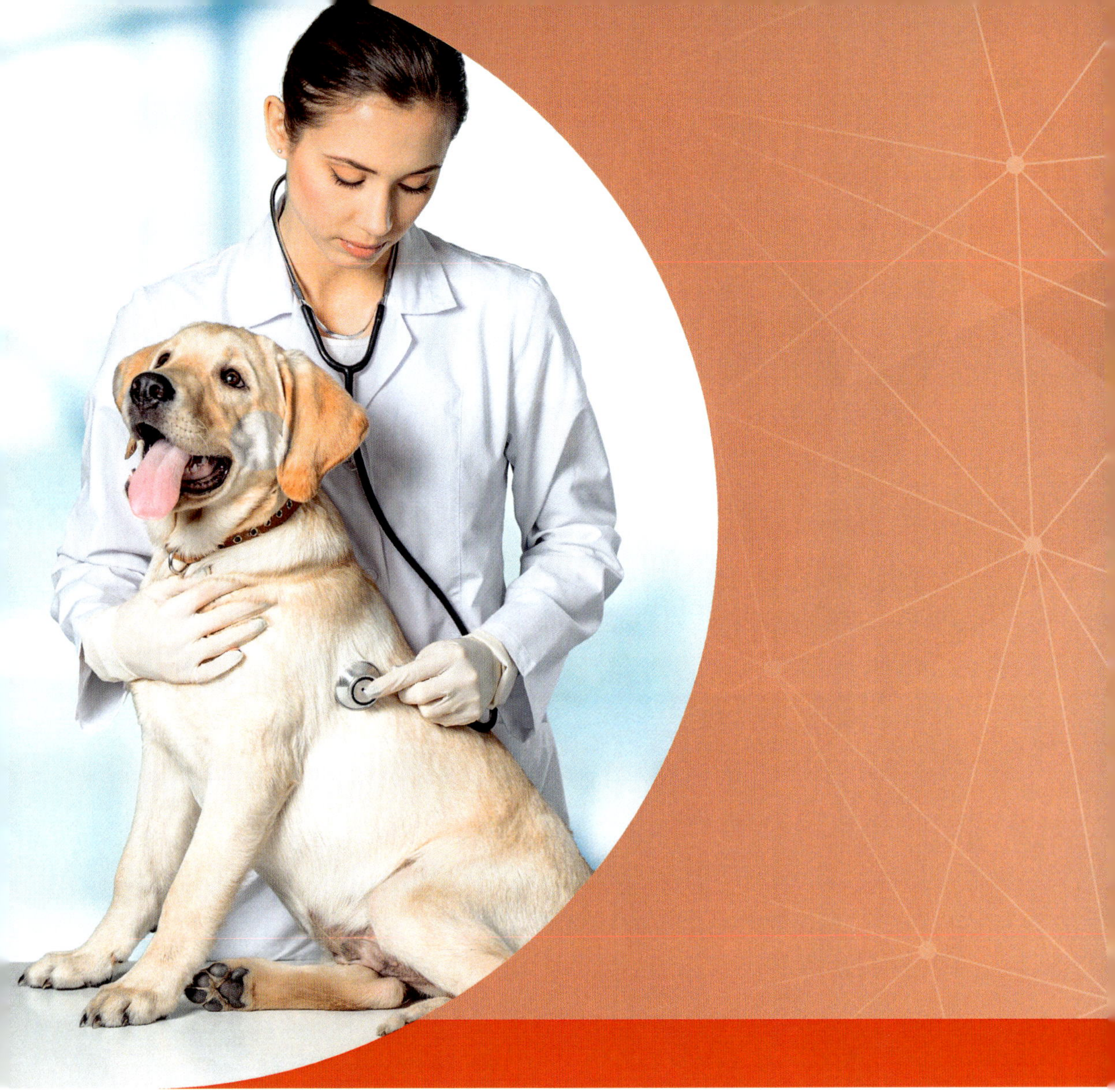

3

DIAGNOSIS

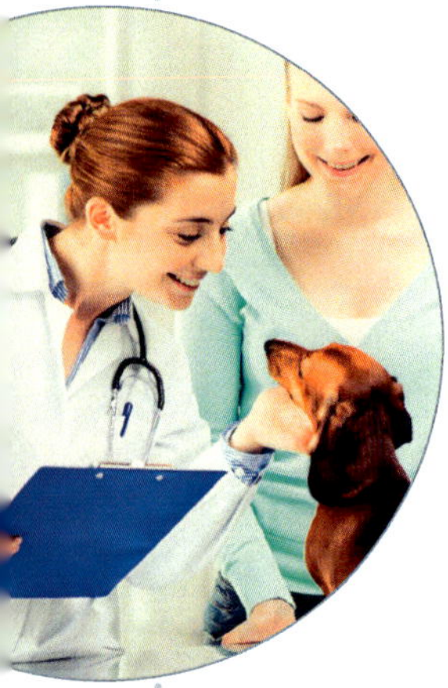

As discussed in the previous chapter, presumptive diagnosis of CVD is generally quick and simple: auscultation of a systolic murmur, louder on the left near the point of maximum impulse, in a small, elderly dog that is asymptomatic or has a cough or breathing difficulties.

The truly complicated task is confirming that the cough and respiratory distress are truly due to CVD rather than another cardiac or noncardiac pathology. In this author's opinion, this is the main challenge that primary care vets face in cardiology.

Clinically, it is important to be able to identify CVD, but the greater question is whether CVD-induced CHF is the true cause of the clinical signs.

Paradoxically, an apparently simple CVD diagnosis based on auscultation and a history of cough and dyspnoea often leads the clinician to make diagnostic errors.

As the end of this chapter shows, signs of CVD overlap extensively with those of respiratory disease; the characteristic signs of both are cough and respiratory distress (Fig. 1).

Thus, when faced with a patient with cough or respiratory distress that may have CVD, these five questions are critical to address:

- Is it CVD?
- Are there signs of CHF?
- Is there cardiomegaly?
- Is CHF the cause of the clinical signs?
- Could another disease be partially or totally responsible for the clinical signs?

If the veterinary clinician can adequately answer these questions based on the diagnostic methods in this chapter, then the options in Table 1 are available.

Patients in Group 1 should not pose any challenge to the clinician: a dog with cough and dyspnoea, without a murmur, cardiomegaly or signs of CHF in diagnostic tests, has some type of respiratory disease.

The difficulty lies in the remaining cases, in which the auscultation of a murmur can lead to a misdiagnosis. Dogs with CVD can remain asymptomatic for months or years, so the simple auscultation of a murmur does not fully account for cough and dyspnoea. Adding to the problem is the fact that many chronic respiratory diseases lead to right-sided cardiomegaly, which gives rise to these three signs:

- Murmur.
- Cardiomegaly.
- Cough and dyspnoea.

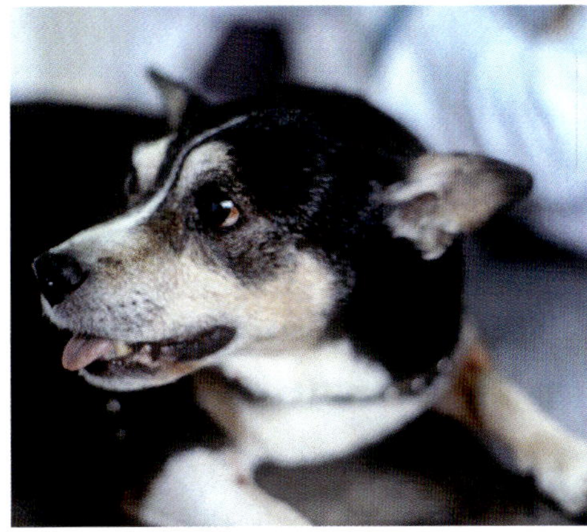

Figure 1. Elderly small-breed dog with murmur, cough, and dyspnoea. Chronic valvular disease is apparent, but the diagnosis must determine if the CHF is the cause of the signs or if the heart disease is still subclinical and the dog has a completely independent respiratory disease.

Clinicians often hurriedly diagnose CVD-induced decompensated CHF in the face of these three signs, when chronic respiratory disease is actually responsible for the clinical signs, a common occurrence in small elderly dogs. Many of these patients thus end up misdiagnosed and, therefore, improperly treated in the subclinical phase of CHF (Fig. 2).

Group	Clinical situation	Diagnosis
1	No murmur, cardiomegaly, or CHF signs	Respiratory disease
2	Has murmur, but no cardiomegaly or CHF signs	Respiratory disease and stage B1 CVD-induced CHF
3	Has murmur and cardiomegaly, but no CHF signs	Respiratory disease and stage B2 CVD-induced CHF
4	Has murmur, cardiomegaly, and CHF signs	Phase C or D CVD-induced CHF with or without associated respiratory disease

Table 1. Diagnostic possibilities based on the answers to the five critical questions.

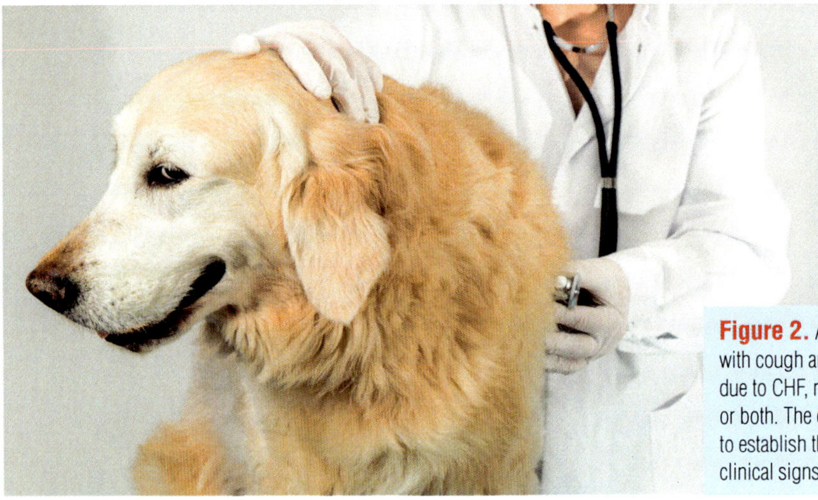

Figure 2. A murmur combined with cough and dyspnoea may be due to CHF, respiratory disease, or both. The diagnosis must aim to establish the true cause of the clinical signs.

In an effort to help clinicians avoid this common error, the following sections describe characteristic findings and methods of data interpretation, followed by a summary of how to differentiate between a respiratory and a cardiac disease.

THORACIC RADIOGRAPHY

Radiography is crucial for the diagnosis of CHF given that it is the only means to check for pulmonary oedema. It is also very useful to assess changes in the cardiac silhouette and size.

At least two views, lateral and dorsoventral or ventrodorsal, must be obtained.

Left atrial enlargement in the lateral view is the most common, earliest, and most characteristic sign of CVD. As the left atrium becomes dilated, greater separation between the main bronchi is seen and the angle between them becomes more obtuse; the left atrium becomes more prominent, appearing as a dense mass superimposed on the caudodorsal portion of the cardiac silhouette (Fig. 3).

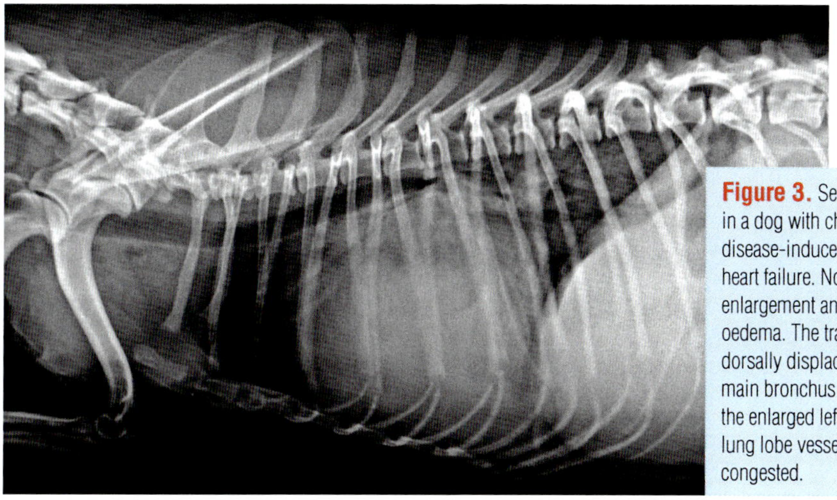

Figure 3. Severe cardiomegaly in a dog with chronic valvular disease-induced congestive heart failure. Note the left atrial enlargement and pulmonary oedema. The trachea appears dorsally displaced, and the left main bronchus is compressed by the enlarged left atrium. Cranial lung lobe vessels also become congested.

In the dorsoventral/ventrodorsal view, the increase in the left atrial size appears as a protrusion of the left cranial heart border at the two to three o'clock position. Along with left atrial enlargement, the left ventricle may appear enlarged in this view.

In the lateral view, the left cardiac border may appear more vertical. The dorsoventral/ventrodorsal view shows enlargement from three to five o'clock, which, along with the dilation of the left atrium at two to three o'clock, makes the left cardiac border appear more convex. Moreover, the left heart occupies more of the thoracic cavity than it does in normal patients (Figs. 4 and 5).

In the lateral view, left atrial enlargement displaces the trachea dorsally at that level, decreasing the angle between the trachea and the thoracic spine such that the trachea appears shifted dorsally and parallel to the spine. The left main bronchus may also be elevated by the left atrium; when enlarged, the atrium may compress the bronchus. This is one of the main causes of cough in CVD patients (Fig. 3).

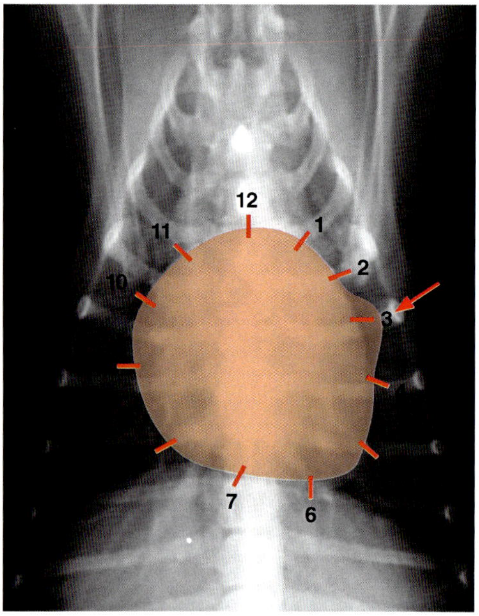

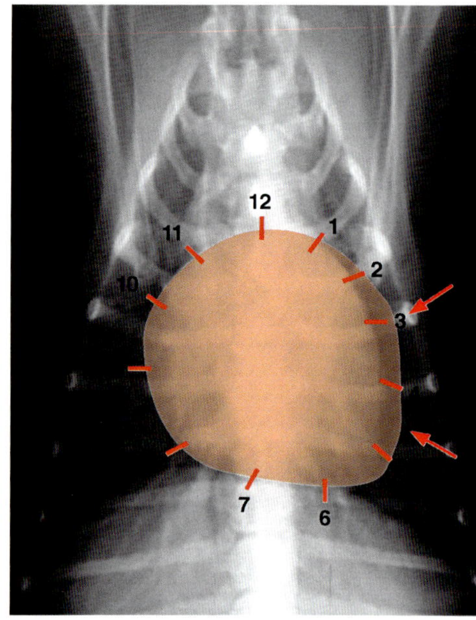

Figures 4 and 5. The ventrodorsal/dorsoventral view shows changes in the cardiac silhouette following the clockface analogy. The left atrial enlargement appears as a protrusion between two and three o'clock. More advanced cases also show left ventricular enlargement such that the left heart appears more convex and occupies a larger portion of the left hemithorax.

> **Thoracic radiography is the most sensitive complementary test for detecting haemodynamic pulmonary changes.**

Left-sided CHF involves the following changes in the pulmonary vessels and pulmonary interstitium:

- As the pulmonary venous pressure increases, the pulmonary veins become enlarged and more prominent. They become larger than their corresponding arteries (Fig. 6).
- The increase in pulmonary venous pressure causes abnormal pulmonary extravascular fluid accumulation. Under normal conditions, the fluid travels from the pulmonary capillaries to the interstitial space and returns to the systemic circulation through the pulmonary lymphatic vessels;however, this fluid accumulates when it overwhelms the pulmonary lymphatic drainage capacity (Fig. 7).
- Pulmonary oedema appears as an alveolar pattern on X-rays due to the increased lung tissue density. This density decreases the contrast between the lung parenchyma and the bronchi and vessels. These changes usually appear

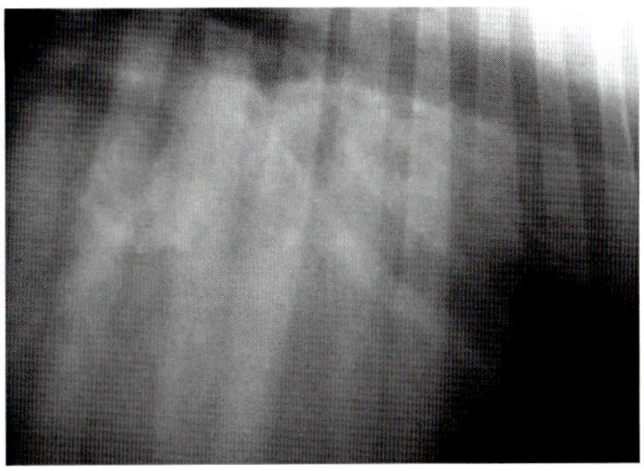

Figure 6. Venous congestion in the caudal lung lobes.

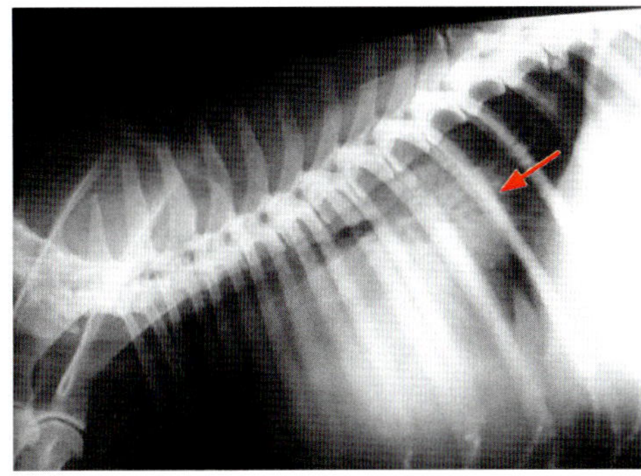

Figure 8. Severe pulmonary oedema from chronic heart failure secondary to chronic valvular disease. Note the tracheal position and the compression of the left main bronchus. Fluid in the airways and bronchial compression are the mechanisms of cough in these patients.

Figure 7 PULMONARY OEDEMA

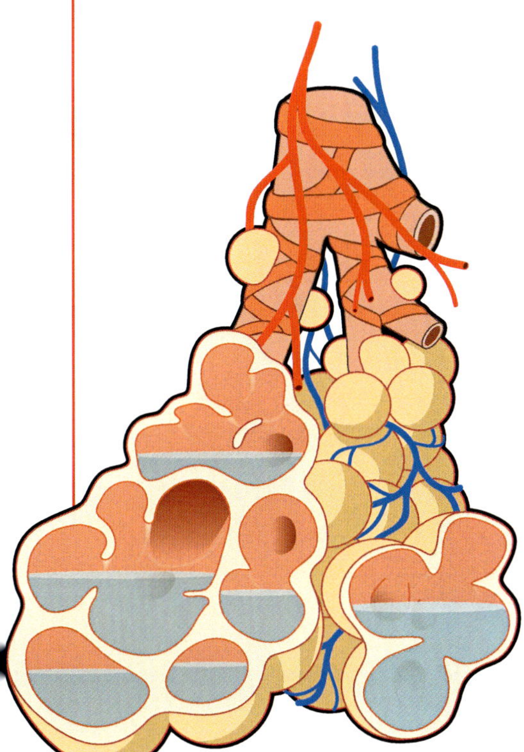

in the perihilar lung area or the caudal right area in the ventrodorsal/dorsoventral view and radiate outwards as the pulmonary oedema worsens (Fig. 8).

- Radiographic evidence of pulmonary oedema is one of the most reliable ways to differentiate left-sided CHF from respiratory disease.

In addition to being the most effective method for the diagnosis of left-sided CHF, radiography is very useful for following the long- and short-term progress of a disease, especially in cases of decompensation.

One of the main features of left heart failure is pulmonary oedema, which results from the increase in pulmonary venous pressure.

BUCHANAN INDEX

In order to determine the severity of CVD and select the most appropriate treatment, first determine if cardiomegaly is present; in other words, has cardiac remodelling begun as a result of mitral regurgitation and SNS- and RAAS-regulated compensatory mechanisms?

Although echocardiography provides more precise information, thoracic radiography is preferred because it is cheaper and simpler.

The most common method is to calculate the Buchanan index, also known as the Vertebral Heart Score (VHS).

CALCULATION OF THE BUCHANAN INDEX

Figures 9–13 illustrate how this is calculated.

1. In the lateral view, draw a line from the cranial edge of the carina to the cardiac apex.
2. Draw another line perpendicular to the first at the widest portion of the heart.
3. Find at the cranial edge of the fourth thoracic vertebra.
4. The long axis (red line) is transposed to the spine, and the number of vertebral bodies spanned is counted.
5. The same is performed with the short axis (yellow line), and the results are added.
6. The result is the Buchanan index, which has a reference value of 9.2–10.5 in dogs.

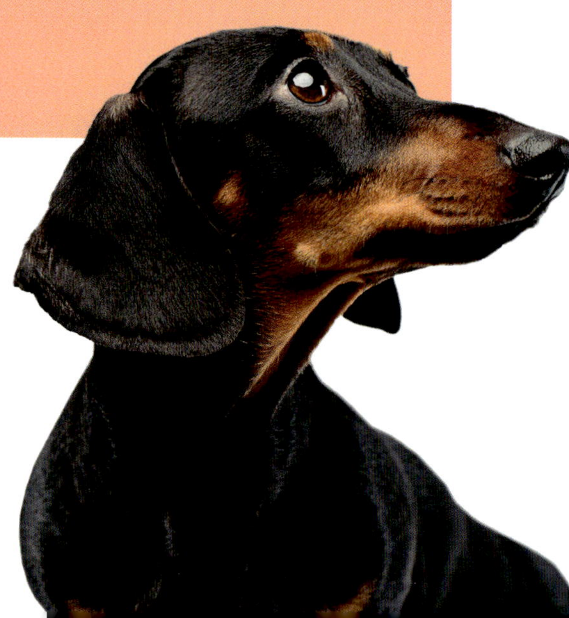

CALCULATION OF THE BUCHANAN INDEX

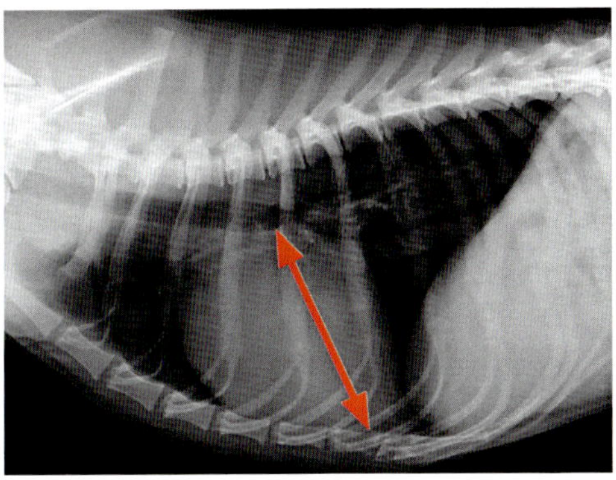

Figure 9.

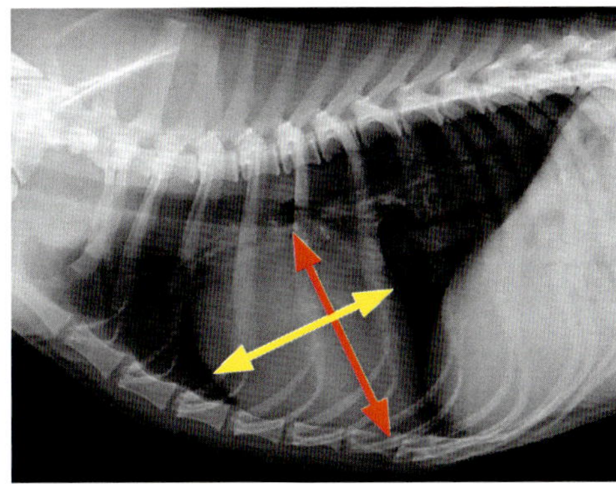

Figure 10.

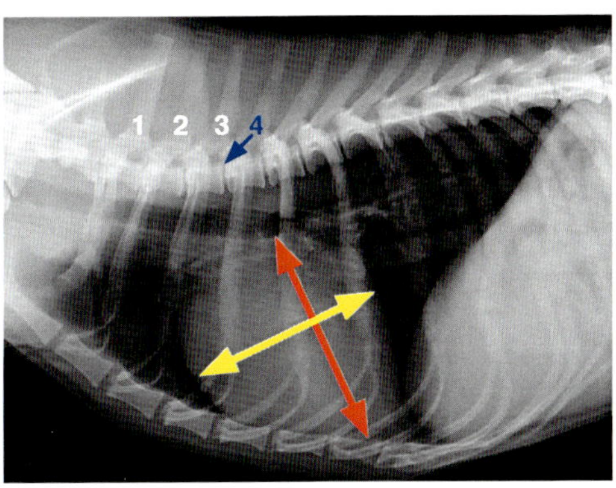

Figure 11.

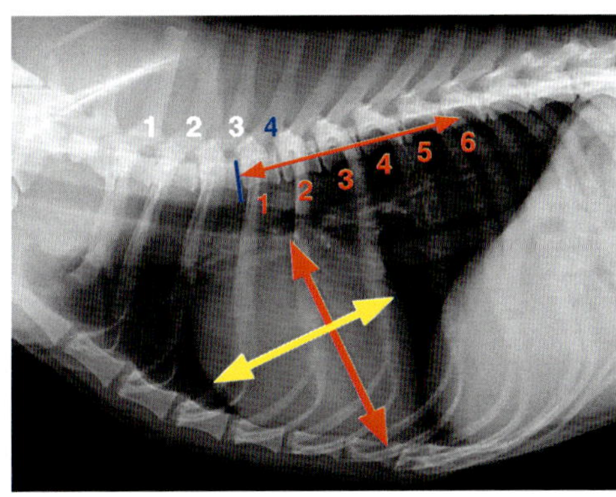

Figure 12.

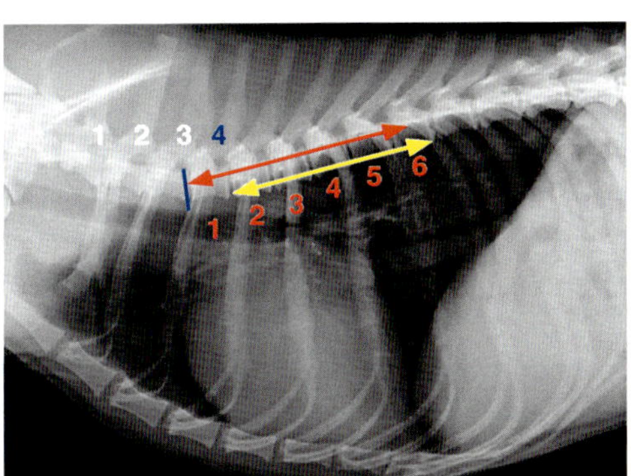

Figure 13. Buchanan index = 5.5 + 5 = 10.5.

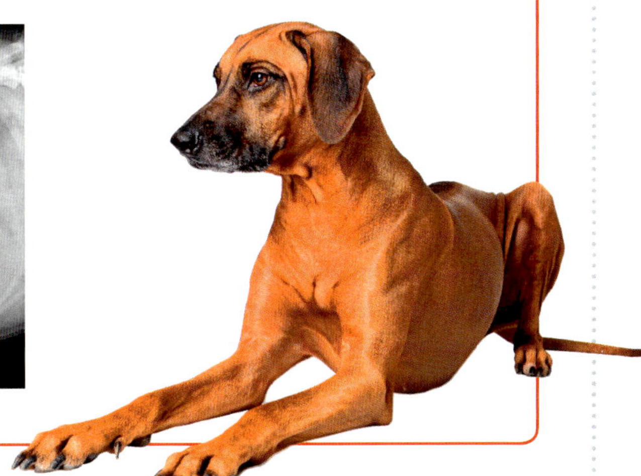

Increases in serial calculations of the Buchanan index may predict the onset of CHF in Cavalier King Charles Spaniels with CVD. Studies suggest that Buchanan index values are constant in this breed until they increase rapidly 6–12 months before signs of CHF appear.

Thus, the Buchanan index is especially useful to monitor the progress of a patient diagnosed with or suspected to have CVD. In these cases, serial X-rays are performed with the same technique (Kv/mA, views, positioning, film developing, etc.) and the calculation is always done by the same clinician.

Limitations to the Buchanan index

The Buchanan index is very useful and easy to calculate, and while it is an objective measure of heart size, it is intended for guidance only and should be used carefully. In the author's experience, its use to detect phase B2 CHF can lead to major diagnostic errors. Clinicians must evaluate this index in conjunction with their experience. Some tips:

- An elevated Buchanan index suggests "cardiomegaly", meaning an enlarged heart. Nothing more. It is not tantamount to CHF, CVD, heart disease, cardiomyopathy, or a dilated heart.
- Patients with chronic respiratory diseases usually have an elevated Buchanan index due to pulmonary hypertension, which causes right ventricular hypertrophy (cor pulmonale), and thus right-sided cardiomegaly, which increases the Buchanan index.
- A normal Buchanan index does not rule out heart disease.
- The reference values are only a guide, since there is great breed variation, especially in brachycephalic and wide-chested breeds such as the Bulldog. Table 2 shows some reference values for breeds with an average Buchanan index above what is considered the normal range for the dog.

➤ An increase in the Buchanan index should be evaluated in combination with other data obtained in the history, clinical examination and diagnostic methods (breed, signs of congestion, pulmonary oedema or left cardiomegaly on radiography, sinus tachycardia, etc.).

NORMAL BUCHANAN INDEX IN DOGS	9.2–10.5
Boxer	10.8–12.4
Bulldog	11.0–14.4
Boston Terrier	10.3–13.1
Cavalier King Charles Spaniel	10.1–11.1
Labrador	10.2–11.4
Pug	9.8–11.6
Pomeranian	9.6–11.4
Whippet	10.5–11.8

Table 2. Buchanan index reference values.

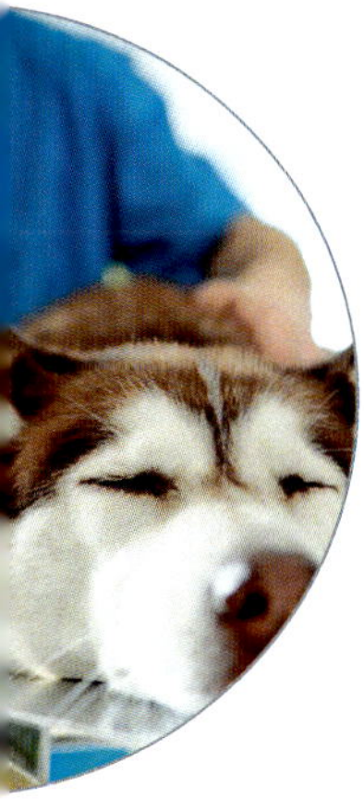

ELECTROCARDIOGRAPHY

The following points summarise the value of electrocardiography (ECG) in diagnosis and monitoring of CVD patients.

1 DETECTION OF ANATOMICAL CHANGES IN CARDIAC CHAMBERS

Electrocardiography is not the ideal method to evaluate cardiomegaly early in the disease, given that cardiac muscle changes secondary to haemodynamic alterations are not detectable until the valvular disease is advanced enough to cause major anatomical variations.

Therefore, wave and interval measurements in dogs with early CVD may be normal even though chest radiography or echocardiography already shows signs of cardiomegaly.

Electrocardiographic alterations suggesting changes in the cardiac chambers and common in CVD patients are as follows:

➤ P mitrale (P waves longer than 0.04 seconds) that indicates left atrial dilation (LAD). P mitrale appears only due to severe left atrial dilation, but it is a very specific data point (Figs. 14, 15, and 17).

- Sometimes, with tricuspid valve involvement, electrocardiographic findings compatible with dilation of both atria (P mitrale and pulmonale) are observed (Figs. 14 and 15).
- QRS prolongation (longer than 0.05 seconds in small breed dogs and 0.06 seconds in large breed dogs) and an increase in R-wave amplitude in leads II, III, and aVF (greater than 2.5 mV in small breeds and 3.0 mV in large breeds) are compatible with left ventricular hypertrophy/dilation (Figs. 14, 15, and 18).
- Left axis deviation is a criterion for left-sided cardiomegaly, but it is less specific than QRS prolongation. Deviation of the electrical axis is more common in other diseases that involve greater alteration of the left ventricle, such as some congenital heart diseases.

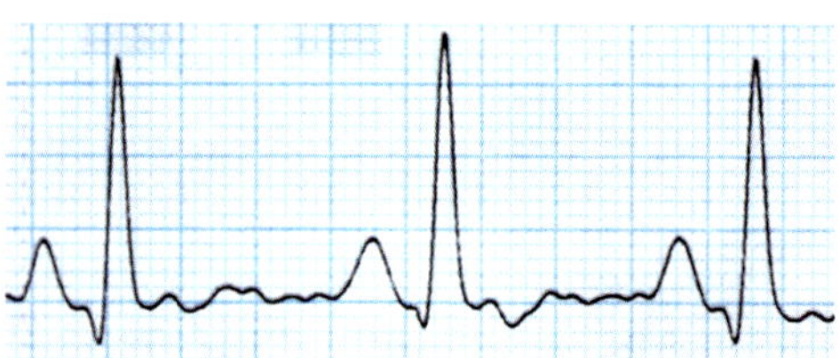

Figure 14. P mitrale in a dog with advanced chronic valvular disease. Wide P waves suggest severe left atrial dilation. In this case, the P waves are also slightly taller (P pulmonale). The tricuspid valve is thus likely to be affected.

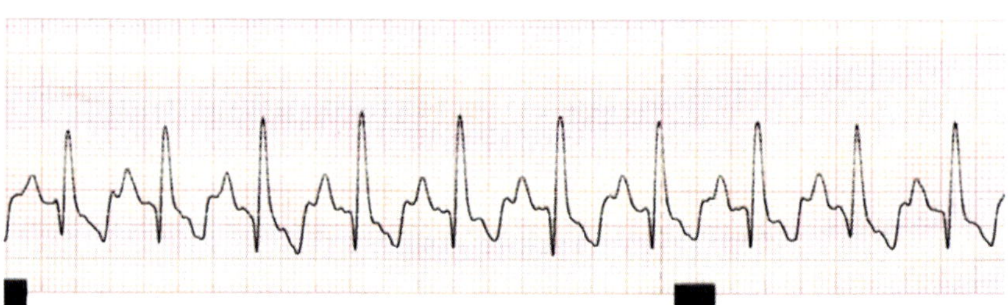

Figure 15. Sinus tachycardia in a dog with stage D congestive heart failure due to chronic valvular disease. The heart rate and regular sinus rhythm indicate the activation of cardiac compensation mechanisms. Note the P wave morphology; wide and tall waves (P mitrale and pulmonale) suggest biventricular dilation, wide QRS complexes indicate left-sided cardiomegaly, and ST segment and T wave alterations are due to myocardial hypoxia.

2 INFORMATION ON THE CARDIOVASCULAR SYSTEM

Electrocardiography can indirectly provide useful information about the haemodynamic status of a patient. Although nonspecific, in conjunction with other data, it can signal possible cardiac decompensation scenarios:

- ST segment changes, especially severe ST depression with a deep T-wave that is opposite in polarity to the QRS complex. If both alterations occur simultaneously, in conjunction with widened QRS complexes, this usually indicates myocardial hypoxia from decompensated CHF (Fig. 15). Note that these alterations are nonspecific and may also appear in other circumstances, such as severe electrolyte disturbances or bundle branch block.
- Notches may appear in the descending part of the R wave, corresponding to multifocal intramural myocardial infarctions (MIMI). They may also result from hypoxia in some cases of advanced CHF, although fibrosis or myocarditis can also be the cause.
- Although not particularly striking, an increased heart rate and lack of sinus arrhythmia, along with the onset of cardiac compensatory mechanisms and signs of CHF, are primary ECG signs in dogs with CVD. Discrete sinus tachycardia with a regular sinus rhythm is characteristic of CHF (Fig. 15).
- As with elevated respiratory rate, tachycardia can be seen in patients with stress, hypotension, pain, hypovolaemia, hypoxia, etc. Thus, owners should learn to take the femoral pulse and record it similarly to the respiratory rate monitoring explained in Chapter 2. Nevertheless, a normal or decreased heart rate with significant sinus arrhythmia in a dog suspicious for CHF essentially rules out decompensated CHF (Fig. 16).

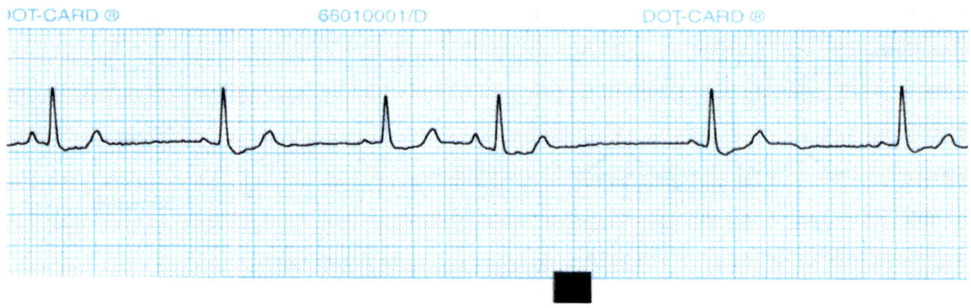

Figure 16. Elderly small-breed dog with murmur, cough, and dyspnoea. Significant sinus arrhythmia with a slower heart rate suggests subclinical congestive heart failure and indicates the cough is likely noncardiac in origin. The presence of an ectopic sinus pacemaker (short P waves in complexes when the heart rate is slowest) should not be confused with premature supraventricular complexes.

3 IDENTIFICATION OF ARRHYTHMIAS

In patients with CVD, the baseline sinus rhythm (regular sinus rhythm, respiratory sinus arrhythmia, sinus tachycardia) persists until advanced stages of the disease; as mentioned, the heart rate tends to increase and the rhythm tends to regularise as the disease progresses due to increased sympathetic tone (Fig. 15).

MOST COMMON ARRHYTHMIAS

- The most common arrhythmias in CVD patients are supraventricular (Fig. 17), most typically atrial fibrillation, which usually occurs in dogs with severe CVD and marked left atrial dilation. This tachyarrhythmia implies haemodynamic instability, so it often heralds a deterioration in the patient's clinical condition. Patients often present with a ventricular heart rate of 220 bpm or higher (Fig. 18).
- Atrial fibrillation is nearly always irreversible, but antiarrhythmic treatment is required. Medication reduces the heart rate in hopes of improving cardiac output, but the increased rate comes at the cost of a shortened diastolic interval; as the heart rate increases, ventricular filling decreases, creating a vicious cycle that must be interrupted.

LESS COMMON ARRHYTHMIAS

- Ventricular arrhythmias (generally isolated premature ventricular complexes) are not as common. Ventricular extrasystoles may occur in highly decompensated CHF accompanied by sinus tachycardia or atrial fibrillation (Fig. 18).
- Ventricular arrhythmias in dogs with CVD are considered a sign of severity and poorer haemodynamic status.
- Ventricular tachycardia is rare and does not require specific treatment with ventricular antiarrhythmics unless the extrasystoles are very frequent; extrasystoles usually disappear once the patient improves clinically with standard CHF treatment.

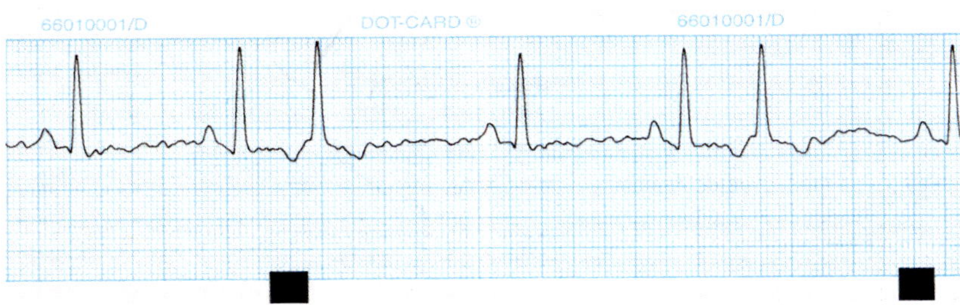

Figure 17. Sinus rhythm with premature supraventricular complexes. Supraventricular arrhythmias almost always indicate advanced primary heart disease. P waves in sinus complexes are wide (P mitrale).

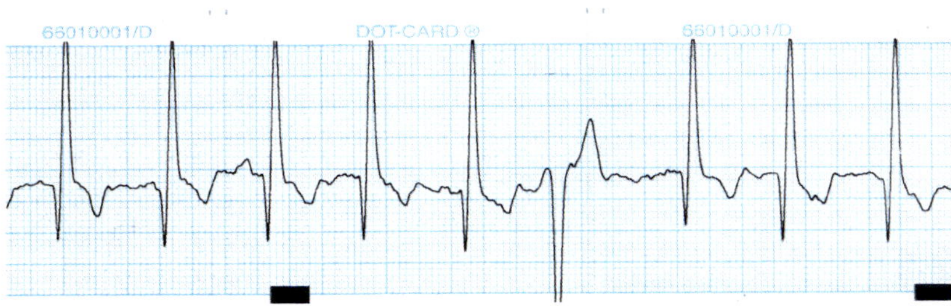

Figure 18. Atrial fibrillation with a premature ventricular complex. Note the QRS complex width and the R wave length in the sinus complexes; these are criteria for left-sided cardiomegaly.

Dogs with CVD do not usually suffer sudden death from tachyarrhythmias, as occurs in certain cardiomyopathies, but rhythm anomalies can cause syncope and must be recognised as a serious complication of CVD to identify and correct.

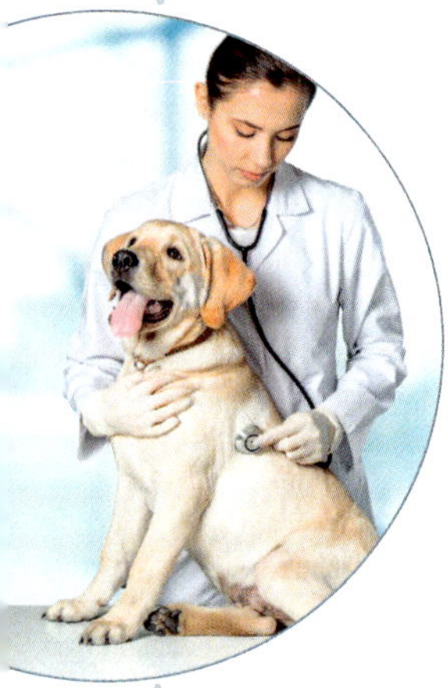

ECHOCARDIOGRAPHY

Echocardiography is a very useful complementary test for the diagnosis and management of CVD because it allows confirmation of both valve deformation and insufficiency via the two-dimensional mode and Doppler mode, respectively. However, it is complex and costly, and clinical diagnosis does not usually require confirmation; instead, diagnosis can rely on data obtained from the history, auscultation, radiography, and ECG. However, if echocardiography is available and the owners are amenable to it, it can be used to confirm the diagnosis and monitor the progression of the disease.

As mentioned at the start of this chapter, observation of a diseased valve and the resultant regurgitation is insufficient to establish causality between the disease and the patient's clinical signs. It is discouraging to see clinicians embrace new technologies while neglecting the basic principles of CHF treatment. The fact that CVD exists does not mean that it is the cause of the congestive signs.

Echocardiography provides very accurate information on anatomical structures involved in CVD and on the degree of regurgitation, but it does not show the patient's haemodynamic status, so thoracic radiography remains the best test for pulmonary oedema.

The greatest limitation of echocardiography, much greater than the cost of the equipment itself, is the availability of an experienced cardiologist to perform the test accurately and reliably.

TWO-DIMENSIONAL MODE

Two-dimensional mode enables assessment of the affected valve and of nodules on the leaflet edges. However, endocarditis lesions are similar and cannot be differentiated echocardiographically. Valve prolapse can also be recognised* and the affected leaflet identified (Fig. 19).

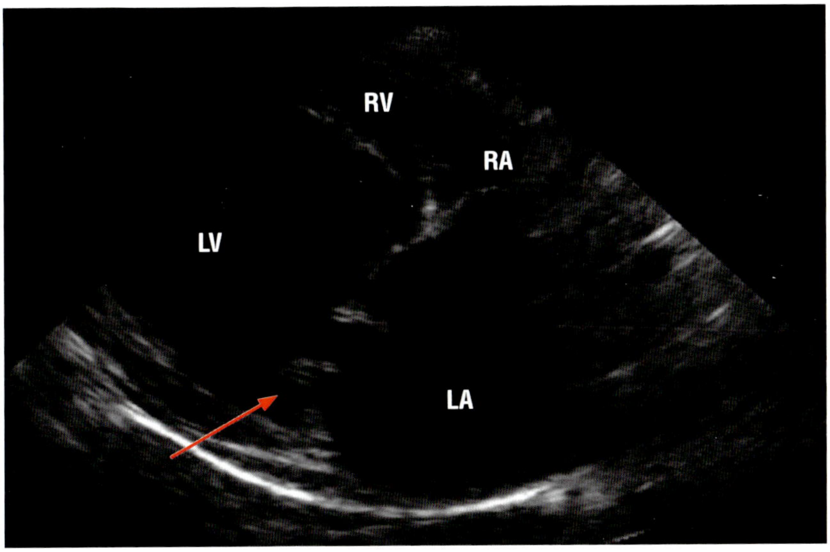

Figure 19. Two-dimensional echocardiography shows the enlargement and prolapse of the mitral valve (red arrow). Note the severe left atrial dilation. RV, right ventricle; LV, left ventricle; RA, right atrium; LA, left atrium.

Left atrial size is one of the most important parameter that echocardiography provides in CVD diagnosis.

Left atrial size is an important parameter as it is usually related to the severity of the process, but sometimes the rupture of chordae tendinae causes acute pulmonary oedema without pre-existing severe atrial dilation.

*Valve prolapse is defined as displacement of part of a leaflet, typically of the mitral valve, towards the atrium during ventricular systole. This results from chordae tendinae rupture.

CALCULATION OF LEFT ATRIAL SIZE

Its transverse diameter is compared to that of the aorta in the right parasternal short axis view during aortic ejection in early diastole, when the aorta appears closed and the left atrium is teardrop-shaped. The size ratio of the left atrium to the aorta should be below 1.5:1.

Determining the left ventricle size is also important. In advanced stages, eccentric hypertrophy often occurs as a result of volume overload due to mitral regurgitation. Despite these effects, the contractile function of the ventricular myocardium usually remains intact, and the ejection fraction decreases only in the final stages of the process.

In large-breed dogs, the echocardiographic signs of mitral regurgitation, along with a decreased ejection fraction, indicate primary dilated cardiomyopathy rather than CVD. In these cases, valvular insufficiency is secondary to dilation of the heart chambers and unrelated to CVD, despite the presence of mitral regurgitation.

DOPPLER ECHOCARDIOGRAPHY

This is a very useful ultrasound modality for evaluating these patients. Mitral regurgitation increases blood flow velocity at the valve, causing turbulence in the left atrium during ventricular systole; colour flow, pulsed, and continuous wave Doppler all detect this problem.

Most animals with severe mitral regurgitation have regurgitant blood flow at 5–6 m/s during ventricular systole on continuous Doppler (Fig. 20).

Doppler has 90 % sensitivity and specificity for detection of mitral regurgitation. A small amount of regurgitant flow near the mitral valve is normal and should not be interpreted as pathological; in some animals, this is a physiological finding.

Colour flow Doppler does not always show the degree of valvular involvement, since some patients with mild mitral insufficiency have a large volume of regurgitant flow. For this reason, the measurement of left atrial dimensions is more suited to assess the presence and severity of mitral involvement.

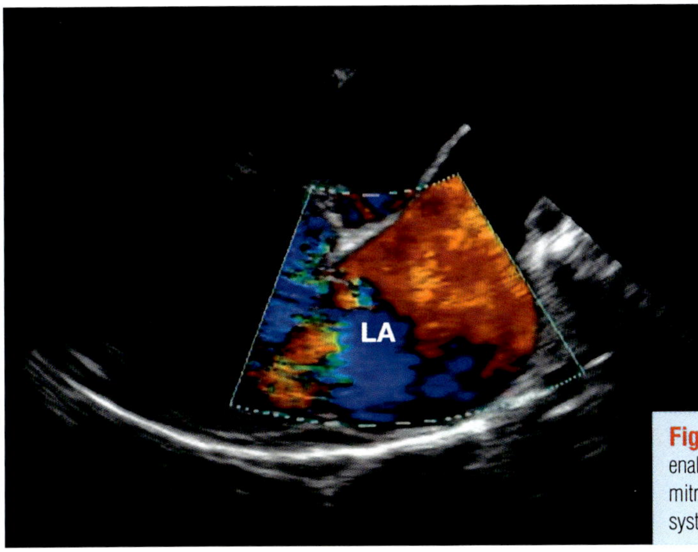

Figure 20. Doppler echocardiography enables measurement of the degree of mitral regurgitation during ventricular systole. LA, left atrium.

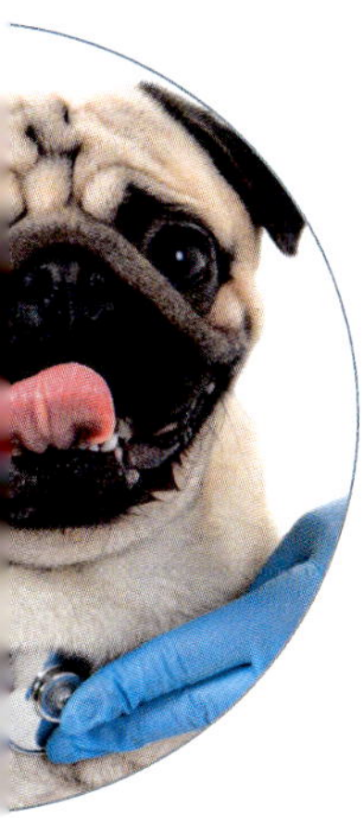

CARDIAC BIOMARKERS

With the exception of heartworm testing, blood testing is not very relevant in cardiology other than for monitoring renal function and electrolytes to assess patient status and potential treatment complications.

Testing for CPK and LDH levels lacks diagnostic value because these parameters are very nonspecific. However, several studies on cardiac biomarkers for early diagnosis of occult or subclinical disease have been published recently (Fig. 21).

The use of biomarkers in CVD is being studied to determine if changes in biomarkers can signal stage B2 cardiac remodelling requiring treatment, as well as to differentiate between cardiac and respiratory origins of disease.

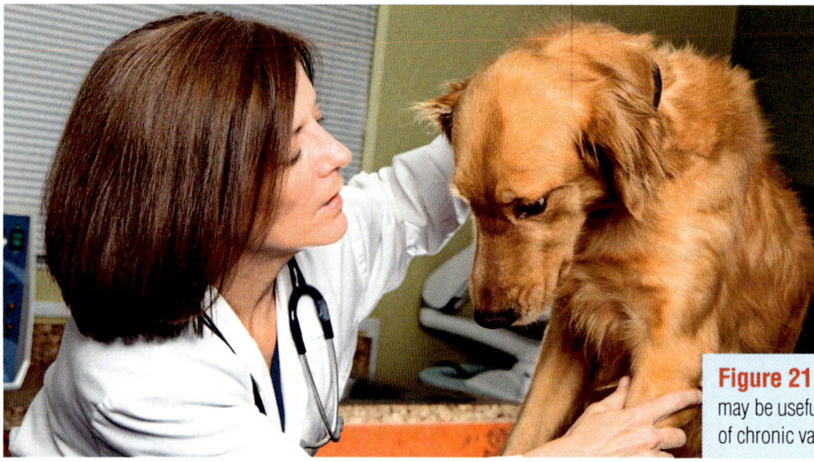

Figure 21. Cardiac biomarkers may be useful for early diagnosis of chronic valvular disease.

WHAT IS A BIOMARKER?

A measurable parameter that can be objectively assessed and serve as an indicator of a biological process. Biomarker tests are reasonable in cost and complexity and preferable to other techniques.

In cardiology, biomarkers may be substances such as endothelins, vasopressin, or natriuretic peptides that enter the systemic circulation due to neuroendocrine system activation in CHF.

The best-studied biomarker in cardiology is the natriuretic peptide NT-proBNP, a neurohormone secreted by the atria and ventricles when they undergo pressure or volume overload. It is a functional biomarker that increases when myocytes undergo stress or tension. NT-proBNP levels can increase in both advanced and asymptomatic CHF; hence the interest in the two indications mentioned above:

- Early indicator of occult CHF.
- Differentiation between CHF and respiratory disease in patients with clinical signs.

The increase in NT-proBNP is correlated to the disease severity, so it may be used for gauging CHF severity and prognosis. However, NT-proBNP values do not increase as much with CVD as with other canine diseases such as dilated cardiomyopathy (Table 3).

> Certain very severe systemic diseases can raise NT-proBNP levels, although usually not as high as those seen in CHF.

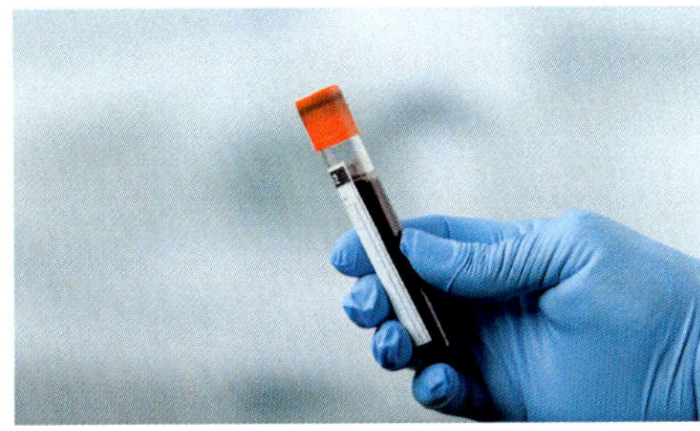

Figure 22. As in other diagnostic tests , false negatives and positives can occur.

As with other diagnostic tests, cardiac biomarkers are not 100 % reliable; false positives and negatives may occur. Thus, biomarkers should not be used in isolation for CHF diagnosis, but rather in conjunction with the other diagnostic methods discussed above (Fig. 22). Cardiology is currently focused on the detection of occult heart diseases, such as dilated cardiomyopathy in the dog or hypertrophic cardiomyopathy in the cat (Table 4).

Plasma NT-proBNP levels	Meaning
<900 pml/L	Low probability that the clinical signs (e.g. cough, exercise intolerance) result from CHF. Consider other differential diagnoses.
900–1,800 pmol/L	Unable to determine if clinical signs result from CHF or another cause.
>1,800 pmol/L	High probability that the clinical signs (e.g. cough, exercise intolerance) result from CHF. Confirm with other diagnostic methods.

Table 3. NT-proBNP reference values in dogs.

Use of biomarkers	
Advantages	➤ Easy, rapid, and accessible test. ➤ Reasonable cost compared to other tests. ➤ Objectively quantifiable results.
Disadvantages	➤ The results are not definitive and should not be interpreted in isolation. ➤ False positives may occur in patients with kidney disease or prerenal azotaemia along with respiratory disease. ➤ False negatives may occur, especially in cases of early CHF. ➤ Early CVD can be diagnosed more easily, quickly, accessibly, cheaply, and reliably on simple auscultation.

Table 4. Advantages and disadvantages of using biomarkers in cardiology.

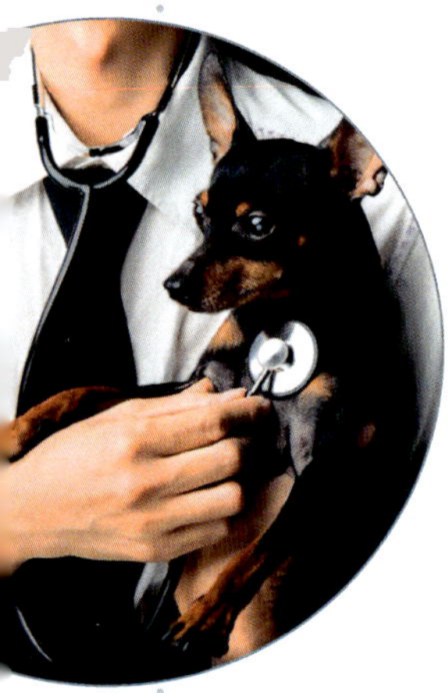

SIX SIMPLE WAYS
TO DIFFERENTIATE CVD
FROM RESPIRATORY DISEASE

Cough is one of the main presenting complaints in veterinary practice. To summarise the above discussion, the three causes of cough in dogs are as follows:

- CHF.
- Respiratory disease.
- Both.

The greatest challenge for the clinician is determining the cause of cough in the third case: dogs with subclinical CHF and an unrelated respiratory disease.

The problem is to determine definitively whether the patient's CHF is advanced enough to produce a cough from pulmonary oedema or compression of the left main bronchus, or if the disease is still subclinical and the cough is respiratory in origin.

This is a relatively common situation in practice, and in this author's opinion it is the most common cause of errors in the diagnosis and treatment of heart disease.

The challenge is to determine the cause of cough in a dog with CVD. Paradoxically, given the quick, easy, and reliable diagnosis by simple auscultation of a murmur, the greatest source of error is to subsequently attribute any problem compatible with heart disease (cough, dyspnoea, exercise intolerance, cyanosis, syncope, ascites, etc.) to CVD. However, empirically this is not always the case, and in up to 50 % of dogs with CVD and cough, the cough is not the result of CVD.

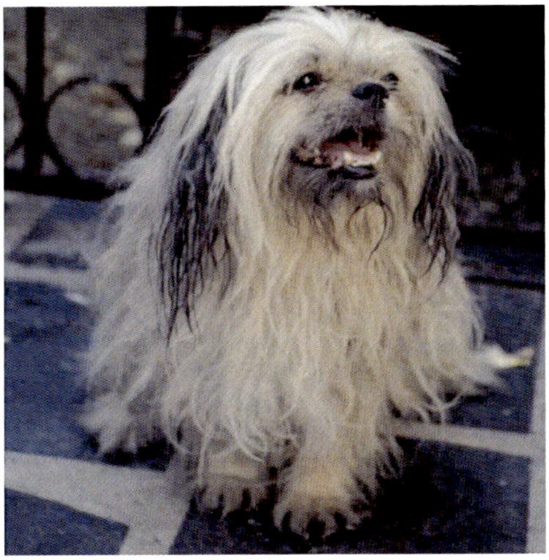

Figure 23. Patients of a certain type are prone to both chronic valvular disease and chronic respiratory disease, complicating diagnosis.

Although CVD is a slowly progressive disease that can remain subclinical for years, thanks to current treatments, even animals with advanced disease can have stage C CHF with few clinical signs for long periods of time. To complicate matters further, CVD patients also tend to be highly predisposed to common chronic respiratory diseases such as tracheal collapse and chronic bronchitis (Fig. 23).

This section provides six methods to determine the origin of a cough in this type of patient, but no method is definitive, and a final diagnosis requires evaluating all available diagnostic information.

1 HISTORY

- Small-breed dogs: always consider tracheal collapse (Fig. 24).
- Brachycephalic dogs: always consider brachycephalic syndrome and chronic bronchitis.
- Large and giant breed dogs: consider dilated cardiomyopathy.
- Young and middle-aged dogs: consider causes besides CVD (except Cavalier King Charles Spaniels).
- Cyanosis: consider respiratory disease.
- Syncope without a history of cough or chronic dyspnoea: consider respiratory disease and other cardiac and non-cardiac pathologies.
- Acute-onset cough: consider infectious respiratory disease.

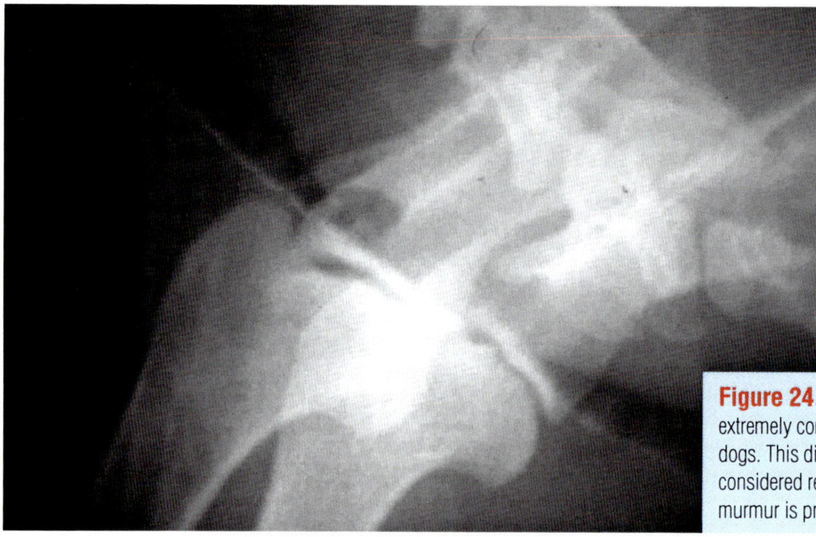

Figure 24. Tracheal collapse is extremely common in toy-breed dogs. This diagnosis must be considered regardless of whether a murmur is present.

2 PHYSICAL EXAMINATION

- The auscultation of a murmur is very suggestive of CVD but does not ensure that this is the cause of the cough. However, the absence of a murmur essentially excludes this possibility: consider respiratory disease (Fig. 25).
- The patterns of the cough, breathing, and pulmonary auscultation are not sufficiently specific to establish a reliable differential diagnosis. Pulmonary oedema cannot be diagnosed by auscultation.

3 RESTING OR SLEEPING
RESPIRATORY RATE

- Sleeping respiratory rate values above 25 bpm or resting respiratory rate values above 35 bpm over several days suggest decompensated CHF and thus exclude common chronic respiratory diseases such as tracheal collapse or chronic bronchitis. Also consider severe respiratory diseases such as bronchopneumonia, pleural effusion, pneumothorax, diaphragmatic hernia, etc.

4 THORACIC RADIOGRAPHY

- Detection of cardiomegaly using the Buchanan index is currently widely used to determine the aetiology of clinical signs. In this author's view, this method may be misused if breed variations and the usual cardiomegaly in patients with chronic obstructive respiratory diseases (tracheal collapse, chronic bronchitis, pulmonary fibrosis, chronic pulmonary emphysema, etc.) are not taken into account. These patients develop pulmonary hypertension and the resulting right ventricular hypertrophy and cardiomegaly (cor pulmonale).
- A perihilar alveolar pattern of pulmonary oedema is one of the hallmarks of decompensated CHF (See Fig. 8, *Thoracic radiography*, p. 45).
- If pulmonary oedema is absent, consider respiratory disease.
- A non-perihilar alveolar pattern suggests bronchopneumonia (Fig. 26).
- A bronchial, interstitial (diffuse or focal) or mixed pattern is suggestive of chronic respiratory disease (chronic bronchitis, pulmonary parasites, aeosinophilic bronchitis, metastatic disease, etc.).

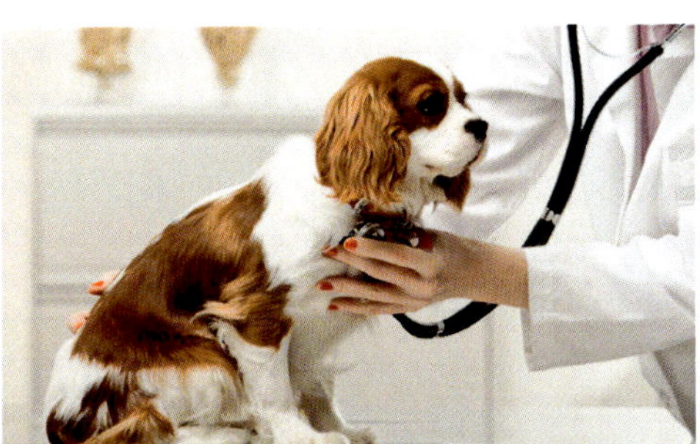

Figure 25. Physical examination can help differentiate between respiratory disease and chronic valvular disease.

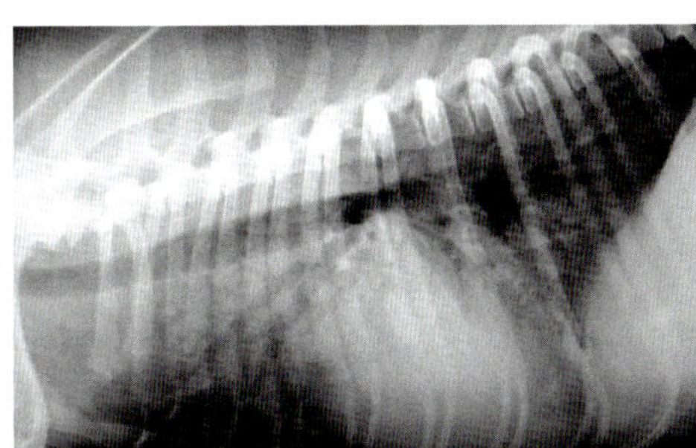

Figure 26. Mixed bronchoalveolar pattern in a dog with bronchopneumonia. Note the air bronchograms in the cranial lobes. Do not confuse this finding with pulmonary oedema.

- If the left atrium is enlarged, the caudal border of the heart is more vertical in the lateral view, and pulmonary oedema is absent, consider stage B2 CHF with chronic respiratory disease (Fig. 27).
- Predominantly right-sided cardiomegaly – specifically, a rounded heart with large sternal contact in the lateral view or an inverted D-shaped heart in the ventrodorsal/dorsoventral view, generally accompanied by a bronchial pattern – suggests chronic respiratory disease (cor pulmonale). Tracheal stenosis in addition indicates tracheal collapse is likely.
- Predominantly right-sided cardiomegaly with a vascular pattern makes heartworm a top differential.
- Unlike in cats, pleural effusion in dogs tends to be unrelated to CHF. Consider neoplasm as the top differential.

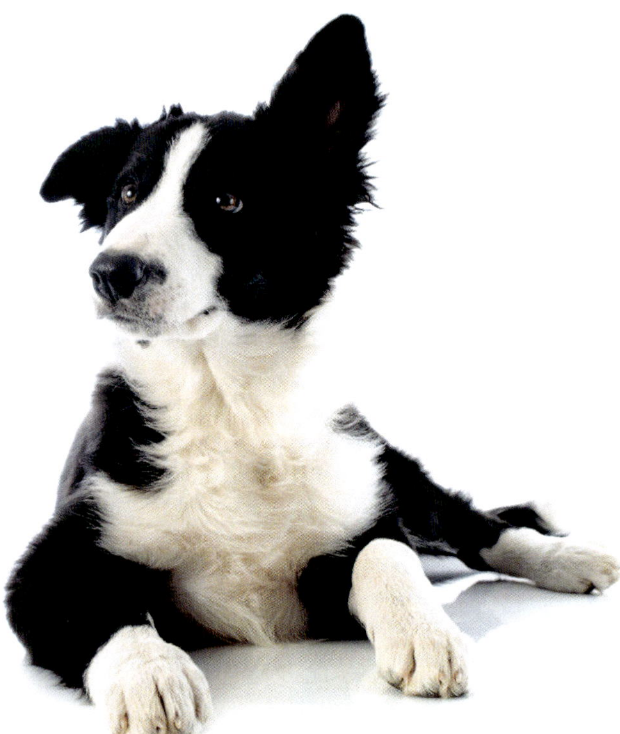

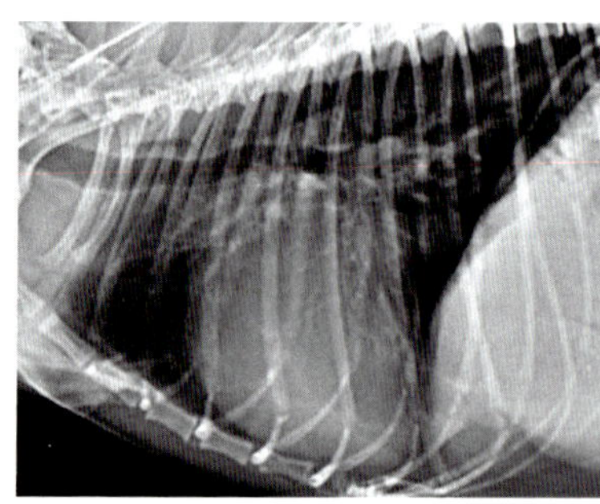

Figure 27. Sinus tachycardia in a dog with stage D congestive heart failure due to chronic valvular disease. The patient presented with a chronic cough due to concomitant chronic respiratory disease.

5 ELECTROCARDIOGRAM

- Sinus tachycardia with a regular sinus rhythm suggests activation of neuroendocrine compensatory mechanisms, but stress during the test can also cause false positives. Confirm the result by monitoring the resting heart rate at home.
- A normal or decreased heart rate with a marked respiratory sinus arrhythmia is very suggestive of respiratory disease as the origin of cough (See Fig. 16, *Electrocardiography*, p. 52).
- Supraventricular arrhythmias are highly suggestive of severe primary heart disease (See Figs. 17 and 18, *Electrocardiography*, p. 53).
- If ventricular arrhythmias appear on top of a normal or slow respiratory sinus arrhythmia, with normal waves and intervals, consider a noncardiac disease such as respiratory disease, abdominal pain, stress, severe anaemia, shock, gastric dilatation-volvulus, azotaemia, or pancreatitis (Fig. 28).

6 CARDIAC BIOMARKERS

- Plasma NT-proBNP values above 1,400 pmol/L suggest CHF. The higher they are, the greater the likelihood of CHF.
- Normal or borderline values do not rule out CHF, but the lower they are, the more likely a respiratory cause of disease.

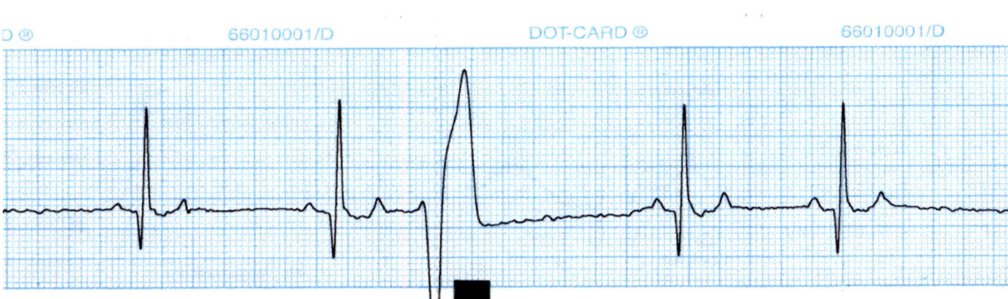

Figure 28. Ventricular arrhythmias are not always cardiac in origin. If the sinus rate is decreased without wave or interval changes, the underlying disease is most likely noncardiac.

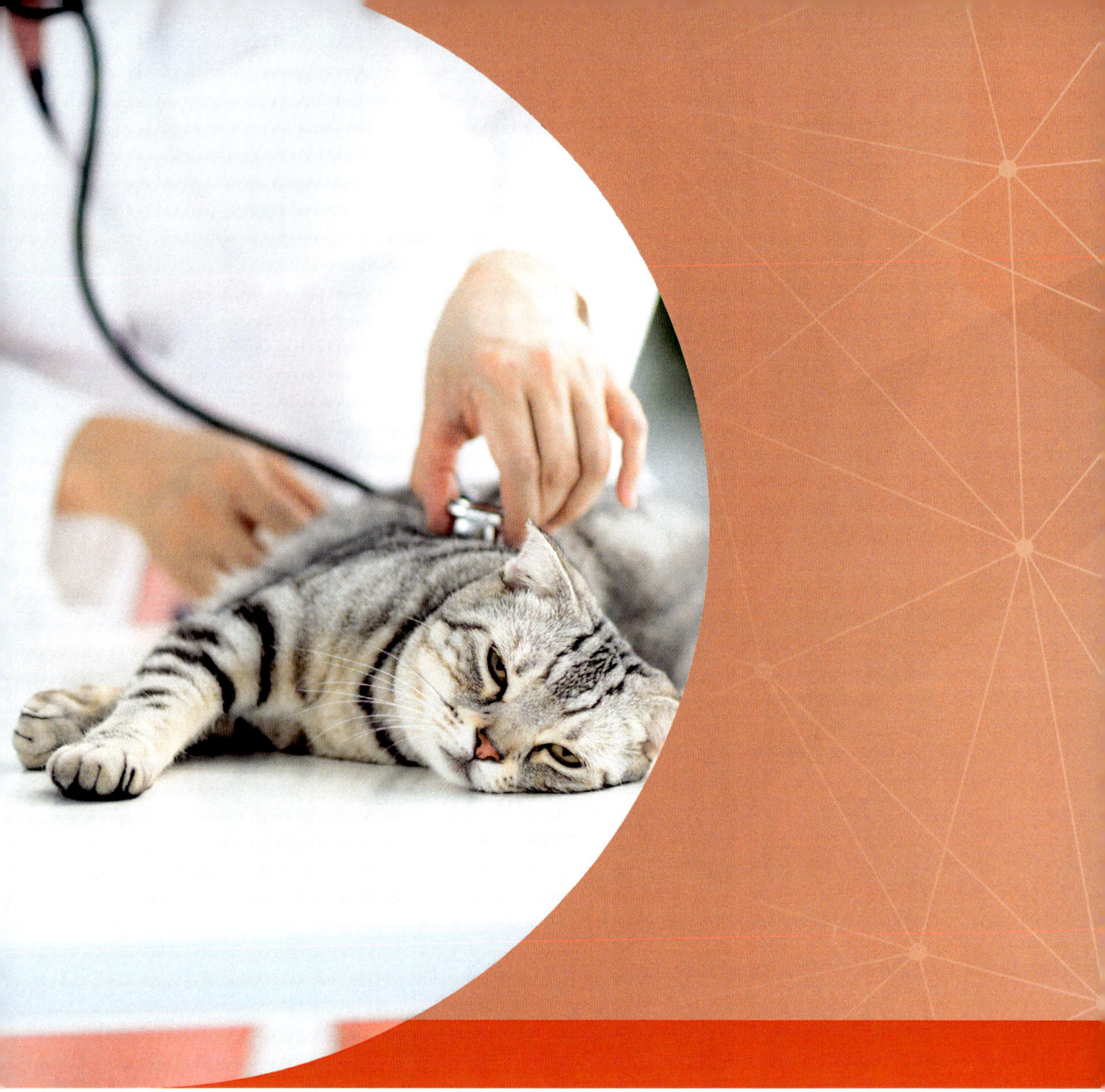

4

GENERAL ASPECTS OF PATIENT TREATMENT AND CLINICAL MANAGEMENT

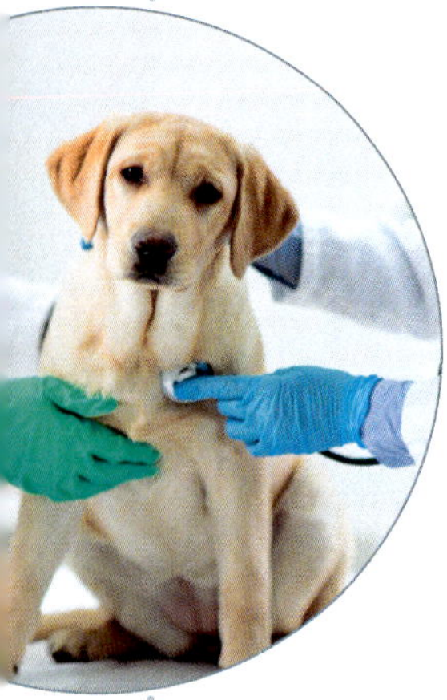

TREATMENT

As diagnosis becomes increasingly evidence-based, cardiologists are working to describe the most common heart diseases to guide veterinary clinicians, both cardiologists and general practitioners. Towards this end, the *Guidelines of the Diagnosis and Treatment of Chronic Valvular Heart Disease* were published in 2009.

This guide, created by the American College of Veterinary Internal Medicine (ACVIM), reflects the consensus of some of the most prominent cardiologists in the world and provides recommendations for the clinical management of CVD.

The ACVIM expert panel established a new classification system consisting of four stages (Table 1).

This classification is specific to dogs with CVD-induced CHF and does not address other species or other heart diseases. This is not a list of inviolable rules but rather an orientation guide based on objective data.

The following diagram outlines the ACVIM's recommended treatment guidelines for each stage, which will be discussed more thoroughly in this chapter and the next one (Table 2).

Stage A	Dogs at high CVD risk
Stage B	Asymptomatic dogs with murmur
Stage C	Dogs with classic clinical signs
Stage D	Dogs with clinical signs and refractory to treatment

Table 1. Classification of chronic valvular disease (CVD) stages.

ACVIM classification	Description	ACVIM recommendations	
		Consensus	Majority
Stage A	➤ Patient at risk ➤ Asymptomatic	➤ Do not treat with special diet or medications ➤ Avoid breeding if mitral regurgitation present	
Stage B1	➤ Murmur ➤ Asymptomatic ➤ No cardiomegaly	➤ Do not treat with special diet or medications ➤ Follow-up in 12 months	
Stage B2	➤ Murmur ➤ Asymptomatic ➤ With cardiomegaly	➤ Do not treat with special diet or medications ➤ Follow-up in 12 months ➤ *Pimobendan	➤ ACEI ➤ Moderately salt-restricted diet
Stage Cc	➤ CHF signs ➤ Outpatient treatment	➤ Furosemide ➤ Pimobendan ➤ ACEI	➤ **Torasemide ➤ ***Spironolactone ➤ Moderately salt-restricted diet ➤ Digoxin in case of atrial fibrillation
Stage Ca	➤ Acute CHF signs ➤ Inpatient treatment	➤ Furosemide ➤ Pimobendan ➤ Oxygen ➤ Thoracentesis/laparocentesis in case of effusion ➤ Sedation ➤ Nitroprusside if pulmonary oedema is refractory to treatment	➤ ACEI ➤ Nitroglycerin
Stage D	Clinical signs of treatment-refractory CHF	➤ Furosemide ➤ Pimobendan ➤ ACEI ➤ Antiarrhythmics ➤ Oxygen ➤ Thoracentesis/laparocentesis ➤ Sedation ➤ Nitroprusside ➤ Dobutamine ➤ Arterial vasodilators: hydralazine, amlodipine	➤ **Torasemide ➤ ***Spironolactone

Table 2. American College of Veterinary Internal Medicine (ACVIM) treatment recommendations for each stage.

At an upcoming meeting of the expert panel, the consensus on some aspects of the guide will likely be modified based on studies published since 2009. The guide has not yet been issued at the time of this publication, but these are likely to be the most relevant consensus updates:

- *Pimobendan for stage B1 patients. One study showed that the administration of pimobendan to asymptomatic patients with evidence of cardiomegaly can significantly prolong the preclinical period.[1]
- **Use of torasemide instead of or in combination with furosemide for chronic treatment of stage Cc and D patients.
- ***Addition of spironolactone for stage C and D patients based on a double blind study.[2]

CVD TREATMENT
STRATEGY

The therapeutic approach to CVD should always be palliative rather than curative, and the focus should be managing CVD-induced CHF with these three objectives:

1. Improve the patient's quality of life.
2. Optimally delay the inevitable progression of the disease, that is, suppress cardiac compensation mechanisms.
3. Increase life expectancy.

1. Boswood, A. et al. Effect of pimobendan in dogs with preclinical myxomatous mitral valve disease and cardiomegaly: The EPIC study - A randomized clinical trial. *J Vet Intern Med,* 2016 Nov; 30(6):1765–1779.
2. Bernay, F. et al. Efficacy of spironolactone and survival in dogs with naturally-occurring mitral regurgitation caused by myxomatous valve disease. *J Vet Intern Med,* 2010 Mar–Apr; 24(2):331–41.

The practical strategic objectives are as follows:

1. Decrease the work of the heart by limiting overexertion to the extent possible. Try to avoid making a "sick" heart "work overtime" to achieve "nearly" normal function.
2. Increase or optimise the heart's contractile function so that it can collect adequate blood volumes and pump them properly.
3. Avoid treatment with severe side effects, ensure that it is reasonable in cost and that the dosage form and route of administration are manageable to maximise owner compliance.

Facilitating treatment compliance is critical to the success of CVD treatment. As an example, a 2 kg patient might need 4 mg of furosemide 3 times daily. If the human 40 mg drug is prescribed, the tablet must be divided into ten sections three times daily. If the protocol includes two or three more medications and their dosing is similarly complicated, compliance will decrease even if the treatment is theoretically correct. Dosing errors, with the toxicity risk that they entail, and poor owner compliance will result (Fig. 1).

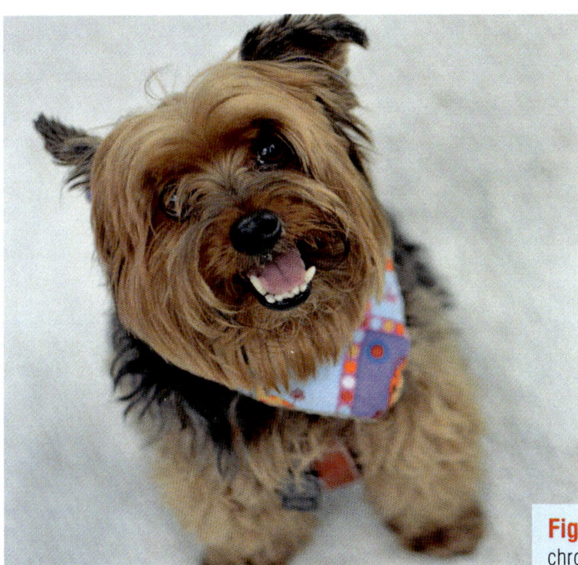

Figure 1. Yorkshire Terrier with chronic valvular disease.

Until the 1990s, the drug arsenal for medical treatment of CVD-induced CHF was limited to drugs that counteracted the clinical signs of disease. The most commonly used ones were as follows:

- Diuretics, such as furosemide and thiazides, in order to decrease the circulating blood volume and decrease pulmonary oedema.
- Venous vasodilators such as nitroglycerin to amplify the above effect and decrease preload.
- Positive inotropes such as digitalis to increase cardiac contractility and boost cardiac output.
- Antiarrhythmics such as digoxin or beta-blockers.
- Arterial vasodilators such as hydralazine to decrease preload and ease cardiac effort.
- Low-salt diets to complement diuretics.
- Symptomatic supportive therapy such as bronchodilators, antitussives, etc.

The following protocols were widely used; many were derived from human cardiology and focused on furosemide either in combination with other drugs or as a monotherapy:

- Furosemide, hydrochlorothiazide, hydralazine, theophylline, and a low-salt diet.
- Furosemide, nitroglycerin, and digoxin.
- Furosemide and a low-salt diet.

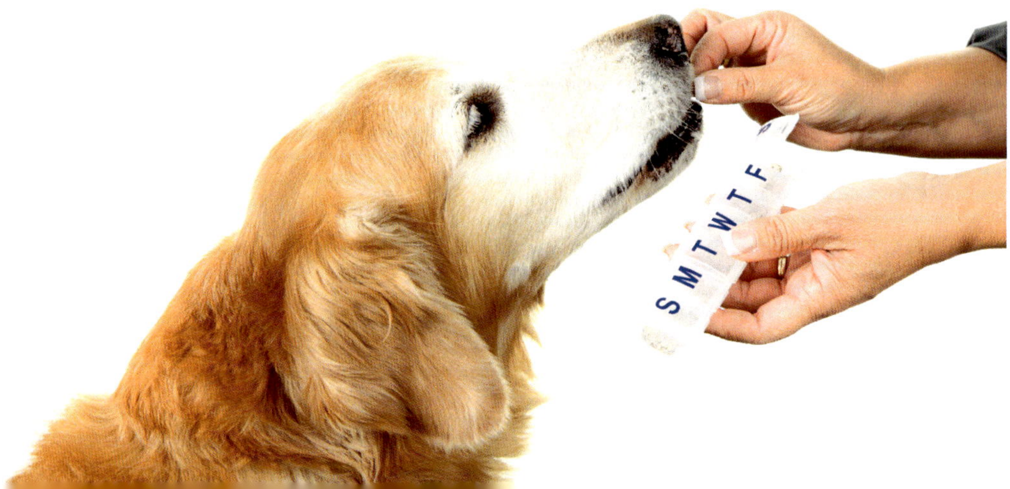

The problems and limitations of these strategies were subsequently resolved with the advent of new drugs and improved understanding of CHF pathophysiology (Table 3).

The development and commercialisation of angiotensin-converting enzyme inhibitors (ACEIs) for the veterinary market, followed by other medications such as pimobendan, spironolactone, and torasemide, revolutionised CHF therapy.

KEYS TO SUCCESS

The advent of new, more effective, safe, and convenient therapies has prompted new clinical studies that have generated evidence for better understanding the disease and the potential role of new drugs in each stage.

Problems with previous protocols
Protocols adapted from human cardiology that focus on systemic hypertension and arteriosclerosis-induced coronary ischaemia are irrelevant to the most common presentation in the dog: CVD-induced CHF.
These protocols had many side effects: severe hypotension, electrolyte imbalances, drug toxicity with gastrointestinal effects, bradyarrhythmias, etc.
They were copied from human protocols, and treatment varied with the clinicians' experience with each drug and the diagnostic equipment available.
All drugs were licensed only for human use and were often hard to dose or cumbersome to give in small dogs, as in the examples of furosemide and nitroglycerin.
Scientifically convincing evidence of their value in dogs with CVD-induced CHF was not available.
The drugs counteracted only some of the harmful effects of CHF; they did not slow the disease progression because they did not act on the renin–angiotensin–aldosterone system or intervene in cardiac remodelling processes.

Table 3. Summary of the shortcomings of the earlier CVD treatment protocols.

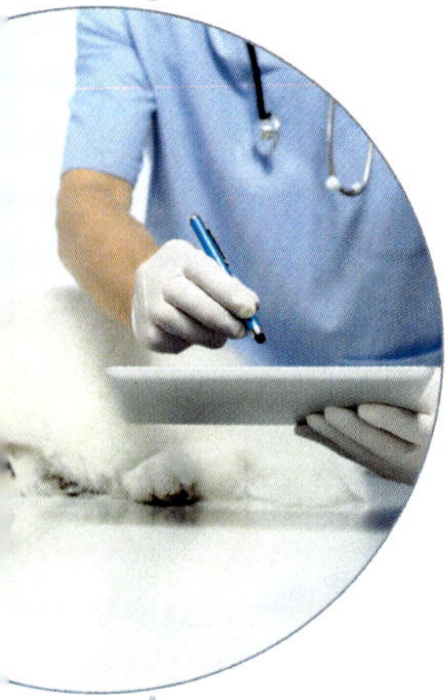

SUMMARY

OF THE MOST COMMONLY USED DRUGS

IN CVD-INDUCED CHF TREATMENT

The publication of the ACVIM consensus guidelines in 2009 marked the establishment of an orientation guide for medications and other treatments in each stage of CVD; these are summarised at the start of this chapter. The next section provides a general update on the main drug categories currently available for treating CVD-induced CHF. The end of the book (Appendix I) also contains a dosing chart for the most commonly used medications.

Angiotensin-converting enzyme inhibitors (ACEIs)	
What they are and what they do	➤ Mixed vasodilators that inhibit the enzyme responsible for angiotensin II activation and thus suppress aldosterone release. ➤ Their appearance marks a turning point in CHF treatment because they block the RAA axis. They prevent fluid retention, vasoconstriction, and vascular and myocardial remodelling (Fig. 2).
Their purpose	➤ It is now widely accepted that the use of ACEIs in dogs with CHF signs (stages C and D) is beneficial for both quality of life and survival. ➤ Their use in asymptomatic animals with evidence of cardiomegaly is controversial. No definitive connection has been shown between early treatment with ACEIs and a delay in the appearance of clinical signs, but some respected authors and cardiologists use them based on personal experience. Studies may appear in support of their use for this indication.
How to use them	➤ A wide range of ACEIs are licensed for veterinary use in the treatment of canine CHF, including enalapril, benazepril, ramipril, and others. They differ only slightly in terms of metabolic or excretory pathways, lipid solubility, and effective ACE inhibition time, but most cardiologists view them as clinically interchangeable and choose primarily based on ease of administration and dosing, taking into account the various dosage forms available. ➤ Once an ACEI is started, it is given for the rest of the patient's life.
Precautions	➤ ACEIs are relatively safe medications with few adverse effects. ➤ Cases of hypotension and electrolyte imbalance have been reported. ➤ ACEIs should be used carefully in dogs with kidney disease, and renal function should be checked before and during administration every 3–6 months.

Figure 2 MECHANISM OF ACTION OF ACEIs ON THE RAAS

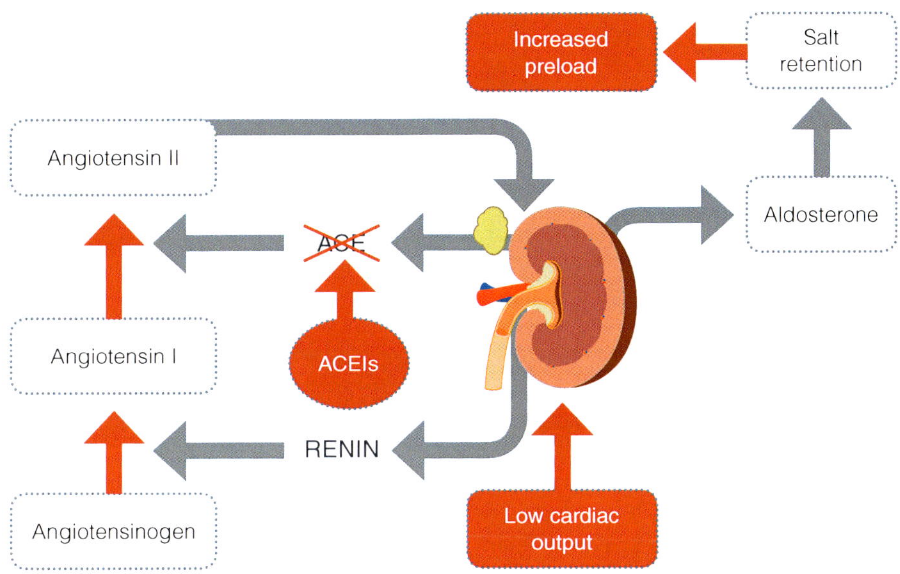

Figure 3 MECHANISM OF ACTION OF DIURETICS ON THE RAAS

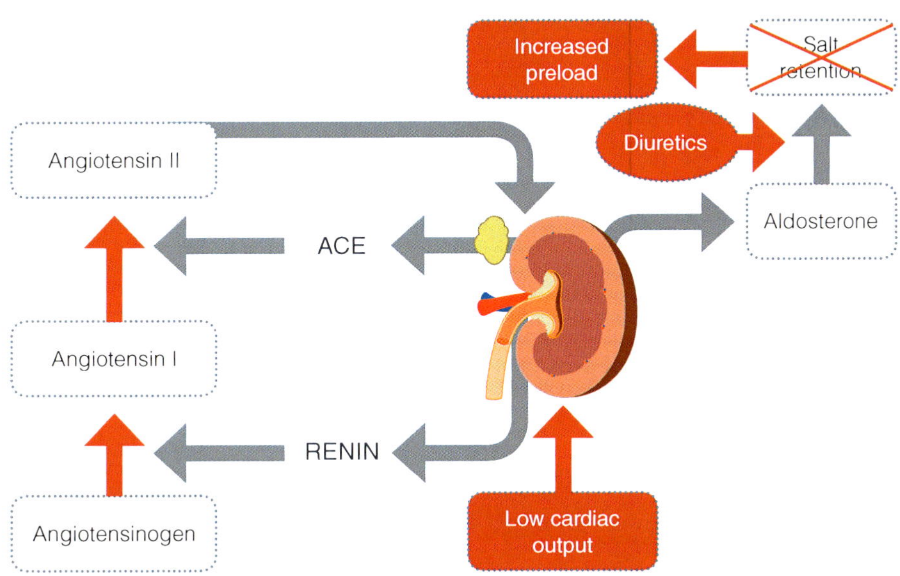

ACE, angiotensin-converting enzyme; ACEIs: angiotensin-converting enzyme inhibitors; RAAS: renin–angiotensin–aldosterone system.

Diuretics	
What they are and what they do	➤ They act on the nephron to eliminate water and decrease the volume of circulating blood (preload). The diuretics of interest are loop, or high-ceiling, diuretics such as furosemide or torasemide; they act on the ascending loop of Henle, an area of the proximal nephron where the majority of the water is reabsorbed (Fig. 3). ➤ Loop diuretics prevent the reabsorption of sodium, which causes water loss, diuresis, and a resulting decrease in circulatory volume.
Their purpose	➤ Loop diuretics are essential for treatment of CVD-induced CHF in dogs with advanced disease (stages C and D). Furosemide is the most important drug for decreasing pulmonary oedema. ➤ Diuretics do not inhibit the RAAS, so they do not delay the onset of clinical signs in early disease.
How to use them	➤ Diuretics should be given at the minimum dosage and frequency that maintain the patient's quality of life and control pulmonary oedema. Based on this strategy and the severity, the dosage of furosemide can vary from 1–6 mg/kg, 2 or 3 times a day, with a standard dosage of 1–2 mg/kg twice a day. ➤ If the clinical signs are severe, IV furosemide at a dose of 1–4 mg/kg may be warranted. If the response is insufficient, boluses can be repeated every two hours or a CRI of 1 mg/kg/hr can be given for up to 4 hours. ➤ Once the patient is stabilised, the treatment is continued orally on an outpatient basis. Torasemide, a loop diuretic alternative to furosemide that is much more potent and easier to dose in small animals, was recently approved for use in dogs. The standard dose is 0.2 mg/kg once a day, with a range of 0.1–0.6 mg/kg once a day; in other words, a dose of furosemide 2 or 3 times a day may be replaced by a torasemide dose that is 10 times lower once a day. ➤ Recent literature suggests that the replacement of furosemide with torasemide is safe and effective and can enhance quality of life and life expectancy in dogs with advanced CHF that is refractory to furosemide, as described in greater detail in Chapter 5.
Precautions	➤ Potential adverse effects of loop diuretics (dehydration, hypotension, hypokalaemia, azotaemia, or decreased cardiac output) correlate in incidence and severity to drug dose and frequency. ➤ Diuretics are not currently recommended in patients without clinical signs (stages A, B1, and B2), in part because they can also activate the RAAS. Diuretics should be started once there is evidence of clinical signs associated with valvular disease, and they should never be given as monotherapy. Note that loop diuretics are essential to treating CHF-induced pulmonary oedema but always in combination with other medications such as ACEIs, spironolactone, or pimobendan. ➤ Potassium supplementation is not generally necessary, even in prolonged or aggressive diuretic treatment, particularly if the treatment protocol includes potassium-sparing drugs such as ACEIs or spironolactone.

Spironolactone	
What it is and what it does	➤ It is a potassium-sparing diuretic, but its diuretic activity is much lower than that of loop diuretics, since it acts on the very distal nephron where most of the water has already been reabsorbed into the bloodstream (Fig. 4). ➤ It is used in dogs with CVD-induced CHF for its specific aldosterone antagonist activity, thus inactivating the RAAS. Aldosterone promotes fluid retention, is a potent vasoconstrictor, and plays an important role in cardiac remodelling. Decreasing its concentration in blood is key to treating CVD.
Why it is used	Blood aldosterone concentrations in CHF patients can remain high even in animals treated with an ACEI, so spironolactone can help to decrease morbidity and increase survival in dogs with CVD by mitigating the adverse effects of aldosterone.
How to use it	➤ Most cardiologists recommend a spironolactone dose of 1-2 mg/kg twice a day along with furosemide, an ACEI, and pimobendan in dogs with CHF signs. ➤ Although insufficient evidence exists to support its use in dogs with stage B2 CHF, this recommendation may change in the next ACVIM expert panel meeting.
Precautions	➤ This is a relatively safe medication, but it can have adverse effects such as azotaemia. ➤ It can cause hyperkalaemia, particularly if given with an ACEI and without furosemide. ➤ Periodic monitoring of electrolytes and renal function is recommended.

Figure 4 MECHANISM OF ACTION OF SPIRONOLACTONE ON THE RAAS

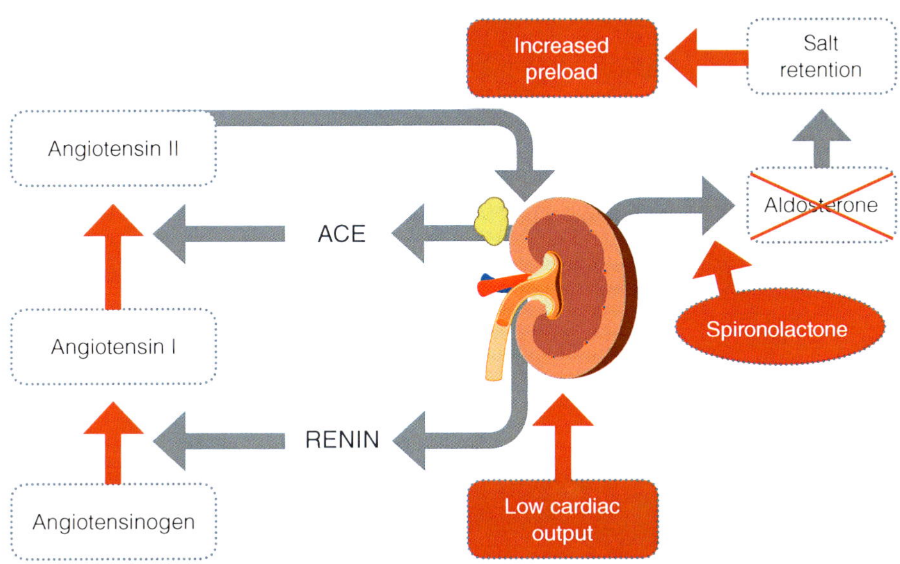

RAAS, renin–angiotensin–aldosterone system; ACE, angiotensin-converting enzyme.

Pimobendan	
What it is and what it does	➤ It is a positive inotrope and vasodilator that inhibits phosphodiesterase III and sensitises myocardial cells to calcium. ➤ The advantage over other inotropes is it does not increase myocardial oxygen demand. ➤ First identified as a drug to enhance cardiac contractility, such as in canine dilated cardiomyopathy, it has recently been shown to improve survival and quality of life in patients with CVD-induced CHF.
Why it is used	➤ The benefits of pimobendan, generally in combination with other medications such as furosemide, an ACEI, and spironolactone, for dogs with advanced CVD-induced CHF are well-accepted by the international scientific community. ➤ The EPIC study has shown that early pimobendan administration in asymptomatic dogs with cardiomegaly who have CVD (stage B2 CHF) significantly prolongs the subclinical period and delays the onset of clinical signs (Fig. 5).
How to use it	➤ In outpatient monotherapy or combination therapy, the dose is 0.5 mg/kg/day split into two doses that need not be equal. ➤ A parenteral injectable formulation is available for acute or refractory CHF requiring hospitalisation.
Precautions	➤ Pimobendan is a relatively safe, well-tolerated drug for dogs, and does not require special monitoring. ➤ Correct diagnosis before administration is critical because a positive inotrope may be problematic or unsuitable for certain heart diseases (e.g. cardiac tamponade, heartworm, and obstructive disorders in general).

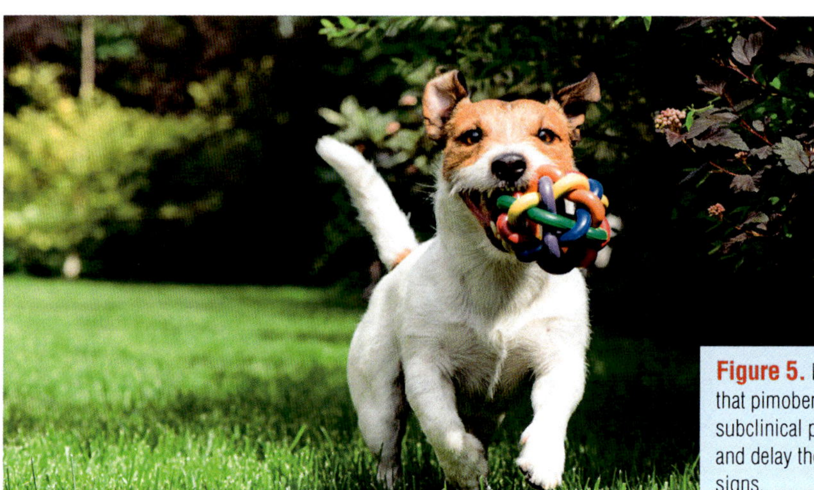

Figure 5. Recent studies show that pimobendan can extend the subclinical period of the disease and delay the onset of clinical signs.

Digitalis drugs	
What they are and what they do	➤ These are antiarrhythmic glycosides and positive inotropes. ➤ They inhibit the Na-K pump to decrease heart rate and sympathetic activity.
Their purpose	➤ Since the advent of new drugs such as pimobendan, digoxin has fallen into disuse for CHF; however, it remains an antiarrhythmic of choice for atrial fibrillation, which is quite common in dogs with advanced CVD, since they usually suffer from severe left atrial dilation (Fig. 6). ➤ Consensus is lacking on the use of digitalis drugs in chronic outpatient treatment of dogs with stage C CVD-induced CHF, but many clinicians use it for inotropic support and to decrease the rate of atrial fibrillation.
How to use them	Slow digitalisation at 0.0025–0.005 mg/kg orally twice a day is recommended.
Precautions	➤ Monitoring is required to avoid digitalis toxicity by controlling plasma digoxin concentration. ➤ After 1–2 weeks of treatment, a blood sample should be collected 8 hours after the last administration. ➤ Blood digoxin concentrations should remain between 0.8 and 1.5 µg/ml. Although the margin of safety is relatively wide, higher blood digoxin concentrations rarely offer an improved therapeutic effect while significantly increasing the risk of toxicity.

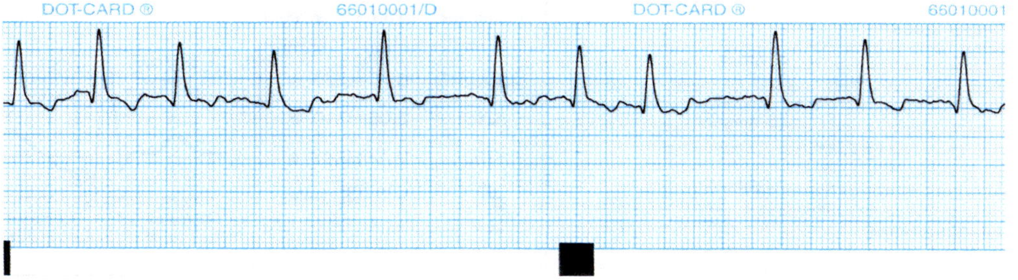

Figure 6. Digitalis drugs remain the antiarrhythmics of choice for treating atrial fibrillation, one of the most common and severe complications in dogs with advanced chronic valvular disease.

Beta-blockers	
What they are and what they do	➤ These are antiarrhythmics that inhibit SNS actions on the cardiovascular system. In addition to their antiarrhythmic effect, they lower the heart rate. They are negative inotropes and antihypertensive drugs. Their effects depend on which receptors they block. ➤ Selective (β1): atenolol. ➤ Nonselective (β1 and β2): propranolol, sotalol. ➤ Mixed (β1 and α1): carvedilol.
Their purpose	➤ They are used as supraventricular and ventricular antiarrhythmic agents, especially in the management of atrial fibrillation alone or in combination with other antiarrhythmics; they are also used as digitalis drugs, but they are more commonly the antiarrhythmics of choice in treatment of arrhythmogenic cardiomyopathies in the Boxer and the Doberman. ➤ They are used to reduce chronically elevated sympathetic tone, which contributes to the progression of the disease. ➤ Although these drugs are widely used in human medicine, few studies support their use in veterinary medicine, and they carry a risk of severe side effects; thus, they are not routinely used in dogs with CVD, particularly in advanced or decompensated cases.
How to use them	➤ Due to their risk of causing a steep drop in heart rate and contractility, beta-blockers can produce a significant and sudden decrease in cardiac output, so they should be used carefully. ➤ Begin with one-half the recommended dose, increasing it every 1–2 weeks.
Precautions	➤ The use of beta-blockers to treat CVD-induced CHF is controversial and consensus does not exist regarding their use (Fig. 7). ➤ Heart rate, respiratory rate, and blood pressure must be closely monitored because of the potential for acute cardiac decompensation.

Figure 7

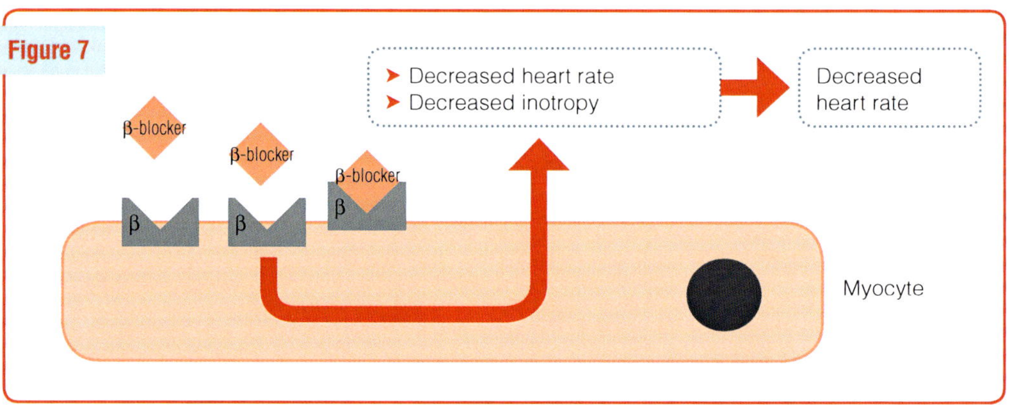

The use of beta-blockers in dogs with CVD, especially decompensated patients, is controversial. The decreased heart rate and negative inotropic effect can lower cardiac output and yield hypotension.

Other vasodilators	
What they are and what they do	In certain situations, other venous, arterial or mixed vasodilators such as hydralazine, sodium nitroprusside, nitroglycerin, amlodipine, or sildenafil may be recommended (Chapter 5 discusses these in treatment of animals with stage C and D CHF) (Fig. 8).
Their purpose	They decrease afterload and preload in order to support the reduction in circulating blood volume and ease the work of the heart in patients with advanced CVD.
How to use them	➤ As additional support for the medication groups described above. ➤ Generally for hospitalised patients with decompensated CHF or refractory outpatients.
Precautions	Most of these medications require careful monitoring with heart rate and blood pressure control, as well as experience with CRI administration.

Figure 7

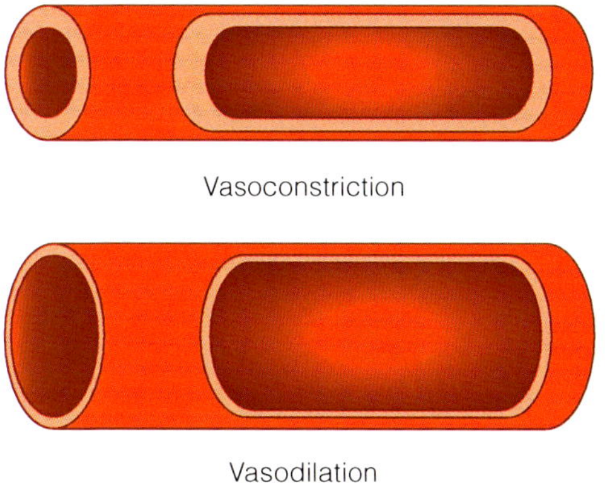

Many clinical signs of congestive heart failure arise from vasoconstriction due to activation of the sympathetic nervous system and of the renin–aldosterone–angiotensin system. Patients with advanced chronic valvular disease may require other vasodilators to reinforce the effects of angiotensin-converting enzyme inhibitors and pimobendan.

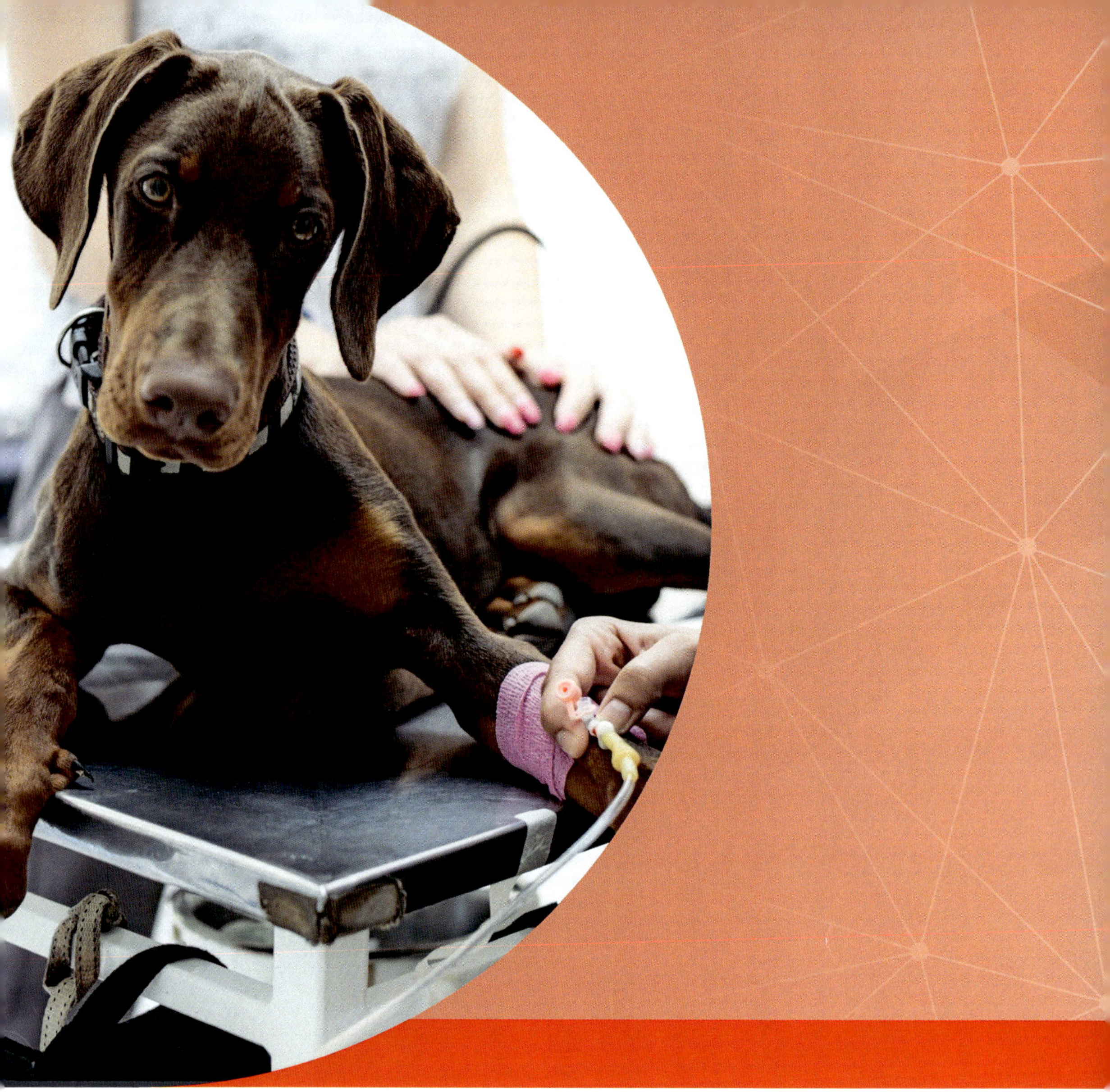

5

TREATMENT

OF CVD-INDUCED CHF AT EACH DISEASE STAGE

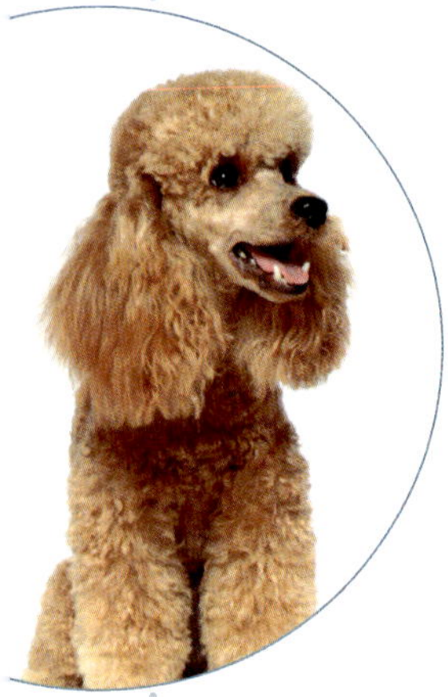

This chapter contains the ACVIM expert working group recommendations (*Guidelines of the Diagnosis and Treatment of Canine Chronic Valvular Heart Disease*, 2009) along with the author's comments from experience and the expected upcoming modifications to the recommendations.

As described in the last chapter, this guide categorises patients into stages for the following purposes:

- To establish an action plan for animals at risk of CVD.
- To identify current or future actions that can decrease CVD risk.
- To enable early diagnosis of asymptomatic CVD in dogs to improve treatment efficacy.
- To identify dogs with CVD-induced CHF signs in order to optimise their treatment.
- To identify dogs with advanced CVD that is refractory to conventional treatment.

TREATMENT
OF ASYMPTOMATIC CVD PATIENTS

Treatment of asymptomatic CVD patients has long been controversial and remains a matter of debate. In the last few years, the management strategy has changed and the current recommendations are likely to change significantly in the next few years as reports appear demonstrating the benefits of early treatment of subclinical disease.

Most academic resources and funding for CVD research are currently dedicated to these patients, with two main objectives:

- Prolong the subclinical stage, meaning delay clinical signs as long as possible.
- Increase survival, meaning prolong life beyond that of animals not treated in the subclinical stage.

These dogs are not obviously ill and lack a structural cardiac alteration. These animals are at high risk of CVD but have not yet developed it (for example, a Cavalier King Charles Spaniel without a murmur) (Fig. 1).

MANAGING
A STAGE B1 CHF PATIENT WITH CVD

RECOMMENDATIONS

- Small-breed dogs that are highly predisposed to CVD (Cavalier King Charles Spaniel, Dachshund, Poodle, etc.) should be examined regularly and carefully auscultated at least once annually.
- Establish a specific cardiac monitoring protocol for elderly dogs of predisposed breeds.
- The owners of these animals should be educated about the disease from the first visit: clinical signs, diagnosis, treatment, nutrition, monitoring, etc.
- Neuter and avoid breeding animals with parents known to have CVD.
- Nutritional counselling to avoid problems with obesity and the use of inadequate or unbalanced homemade diets.
- Do not begin any CHF-specific treatment.

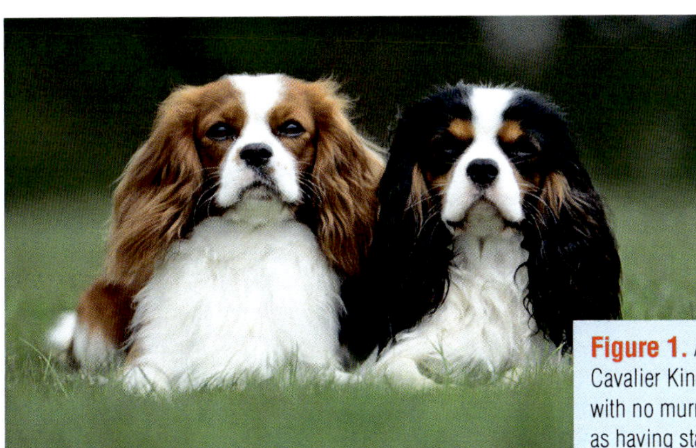

Figure 1. Asymptomatic Cavalier King Charles Spaniels with no murmur are designated as having stage A CHF.

These dogs have been diagnosed with a classic murmur of CVD but have no clinical signs of CHF or any structural cardiac alteration; in other words, no radiographic or echocardiographic evidence of left atrial or ventricular dilation exists and the vertebral heart score is normal.

No treatment to date has shown to be effective (or counterproductive) at this stage to delay the onset of clinical signs, mitigate the disease progression, or prolong life expectancy (Fig. 2).

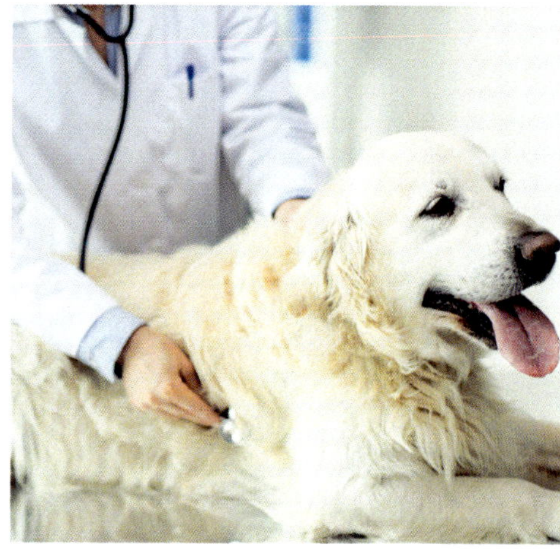

Figure 2. A dog with murmur but no signs of CHF or cardiomegaly is diagnosed with stage B1 CHF. No specific cardiac treatment is recommended.

RECOMMENDATIONS

- Take thoracic X-rays in two positions to ensure no cardiomegaly, venous congestion, or pulmonary oedema is present.
- Keep the initial X-rays for reference and record the technique used.
- Perform an ECG.
- Measure the blood pressure.
- Perform an echocardiogram if the auscultation findings or the X-rays are atypical or inconclusive.
- Perform an echocardiogram in large breed dogs to rule out a congenital disease and dilated cardiomyopathy as causes of murmur.
- Baseline blood work.
- Full cardiac examination every 6–12 months.
- Neuter or avoid breeding young Cavalier King Charles Spaniels and individuals of other predisposed breeds with murmurs.
- Nutritional counselling to avoid problems with obesity and the use of inadequate or unbalanced homemade diets.
- Correct unbalanced diets and recommend controlled weight loss in obese patients.
- Do not begin any disease-specific treatment.

MANAGING
A STAGE B2 CHF PATIENT WITH CVD

These dogs have a classic CVD murmur but have never manifested clinical signs of CHF; they have clear radiographic or echocardiographic evidence of cardiac remodelling (dilated left atrium, left ventricle, or both).

Treatment of these patients is controversial and expert treatment criteria differ, with insufficient scientific evidence to reach consensus on a treatment model. The recent EPIC study supports the use of pimobendan at this stage for its proven ability to significantly prolong the subclinical period (Fig. 3).

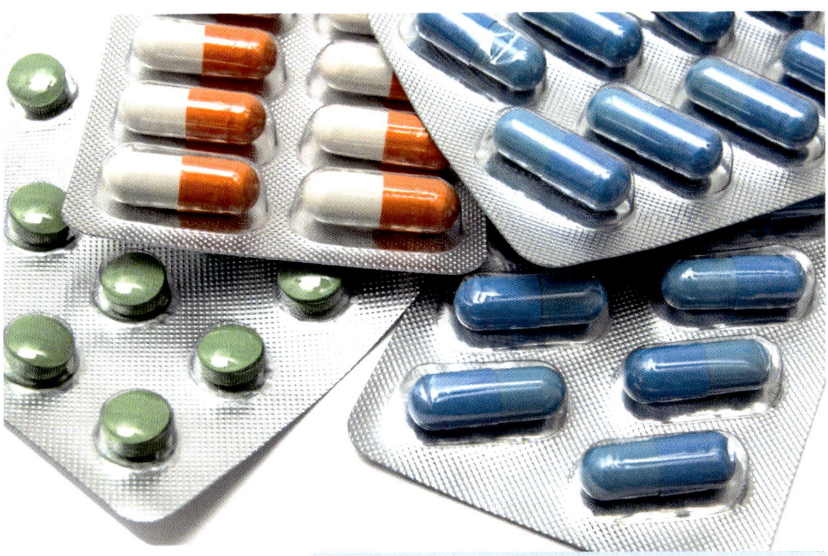

Figure 3. Recent studies have explored the efficacy of pimobendan in dogs with stage B2 CVD-induced CHF to delay the onset of clinical signs.

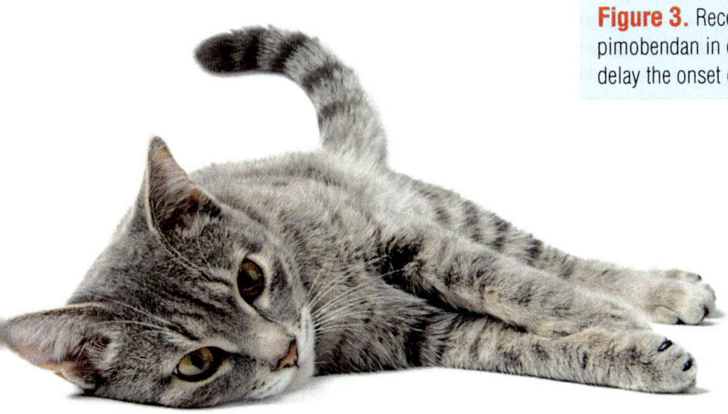

RECOMMENDATIONS

- Pimobendan, 0.25 mg/kg orally twice a day.

  The EPIC study showed a 15-month extension of the subclinical period in dogs with stage B2 CVD-induced CHF treated with pimobendan compared to placebo. This study was published after the ACVIM guidelines. The 2009 recommendations are likely to be reviewed in 2018, and a majority or a consensus is likely to recommend pimobendan at this stage. Until then, the clinician must choose whether or not to prescribe it based on the financial cost to the owners and the fact that cardiomegaly should be evident in order to initiate therapy. Pimobendan is considered safe and does not require close monitoring, so the benefit:risk ratio seems to favour its use.
- An ACEI orally at the standard dose.

  Most cardiologists recommend starting treatment with an ACEI despite the fact that studies at this stage are inconclusive and have not demonstrated a statistically significant delay in the progression of CHF. Since the publication of the EPIC study, the benefits of coadministration of pimobendan plus an ACEI have not been demonstrated.

  Although ACEIs have proven very effective in the treatment of CVD with advanced CHF, their potential side effects warrant use with discretion at this stage of the disease until new studies are performed.
- While some cardiologists use spironolactone, little evidence exists that adding it to an ACEI or pimobendan has any positive effect at this stage. The commercial formulation that combines spironolactone with benazepril should be used at the clinician's discretion.
- Loop diuretics: no evidence of benefit at this stage is available, and they may activate the RAAS. Their use is discouraged.
- Some cardiologists recommend the use of beta-blockers (atenolol, carvedilol) or calcium channel blockers (amlodipine) in these stages, particularly when evidence of significant cardiac remodelling exists. The lack of evidence of benefit, the potential side effects, and the need for more comprehensive ECG and blood pressure monitoring are the reasons this author does not use them.
- A balanced, palatable diet or one moderately restricted in salt.
- A controlled weight loss programme in obese patients.

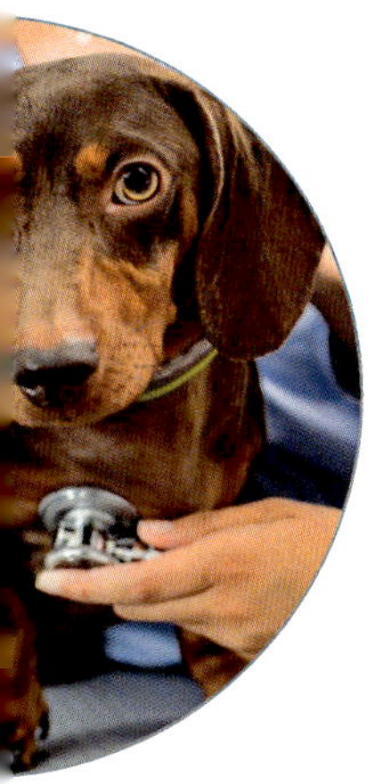

TREATMENT
OF PATIENTS
WITH ADVANCED CVD-INDUCED CHF

A diagnosis of stage C or D CVD-induced CHF requires fulfilling four criteria:

- Auscultation of a murmur.
- Evidence of cardiac remodelling.
- Identification of CHF signs.
- Evidence that clinical signs are the result of CHF.

Regardless of whether the patient's signalment is characteristic of CVD (small elderly dog), if no murmur is ausculted, no clear signs of left-sided cardiomegaly appear, and the diagnostics do not suggest decompensated CHF (pulmonary oedema, elevated heart and respiratory rate, etc.), a CHF diagnosis is unlikely (Fig. 4).

In addition to these situations, reconsider a diagnosis of advanced CVD-induced CHF in the following cases:

- The initial, predominant signs are not congestive (cough and respiratory distress). For example, dogs with a history of syncope or ascites but no chronic respiratory signs.
- The response to conventional CHF treatment is not as anticipated. In these cases, the clinician should neither increase the dosage nor add drugs to the CHF protocol; instead, the clinician should ensure that the CHF diagnosis is correct and that no other noncardiac disease exists that may account for the clinical situation.

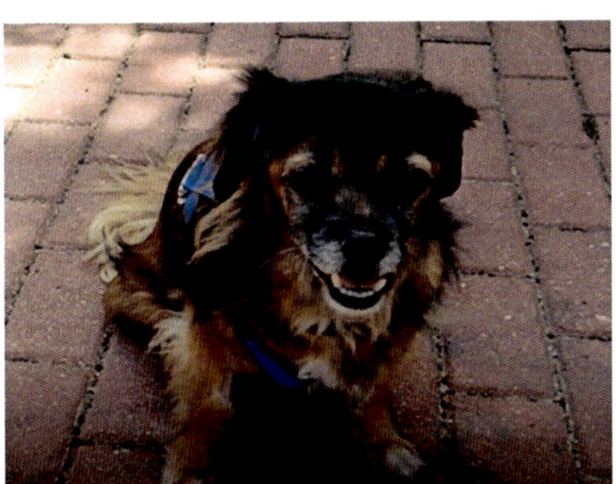

Figure 4. The auscultation of a murmur or the presence of signs compatible with congestive heart failure in a small-breed elderly dog are insufficient to establish a diagnosis and initiate congestive heart failure treatment.

Although the ACVIM guidelines differentiate between stage C and D patients in terms of those presenting acutely and in need of hospitalisation versus those with chronic disease who can be treated at home, it is most instructive to first consider long-term outpatient treatment of CVD-induced CHF (stage C), then outpatient management of treatment-refractory patients (stage D), and finally steps to manage acute CHF that requires hospitalisation.

Because this is the typical chronology of CVD, this is the sequence of the following discussion.

OUTPATIENT MANAGEMENT
OF PATIENTS WITH STAGE C CVD-INDUCED CHF

These are dogs with heart murmurs and structural alterations who have or have had clinical signs of CHF. These signs usually appear months or years after the murmur is first ausculted, and they gradually worsen with disease progression. Congestive signs tend to predominate initially in situations of high cardiovascular demand, especially during exercise, and they begin to appear in less demanding situations, or even at rest, as the disease progresses and cardiac function deteriorates. These animals present with chronic disease and do not require hospitalisation at this time.

Included in this group are dogs that have shown CHF signs previously and have improved since treatment; some may even be completely asymptomatic.

There are six chronic treatment objectives at this stage:

- To improve haemodynamic status (decrease preload and afterload while sustaining or increasing cardiac output).
- To slow down disease progression.
- To prolong survival.
- To reduce CHF clinical signs.
- To improve exercise tolerance..
- To improve the patient's quality of life.

RECOMMENDATIONS

- Verify that the clinical signs are a result of CVD-induced CHF. Exclude possible associated chronic respiratory diseases such as tracheal collapse and perform all the tests listed in Chapter 3 to differentiate CHF from respiratory disease (X-rays, ECG, resting respiratory rate, NT-proBNP, etc.) (Fig. 5).
- If CHF treatment is started, unless otherwise specified, it should be continued for the patient's life. The costs of treatment and monitoring, as well as the inconveniences of administering drugs, are key factors in long-term success. The clinician should strive to maximise owner compliance with recommendations. The long-term CHF treatment plan should always be tailored to the owner's situation and abilities; dosing should be as clear and simple as possible. Select the most palatable dosage forms that are easiest to give and best adapted to the patient's weight, and that require the lowest frequency of administration. Thus, the dose should be adjusted to a quarter, half, or a whole pill rather than an exact but cumbersome dose (Fig. 6). A general rule is that the less compliant the owner is suspected to be, the simpler the treatment plan should be.

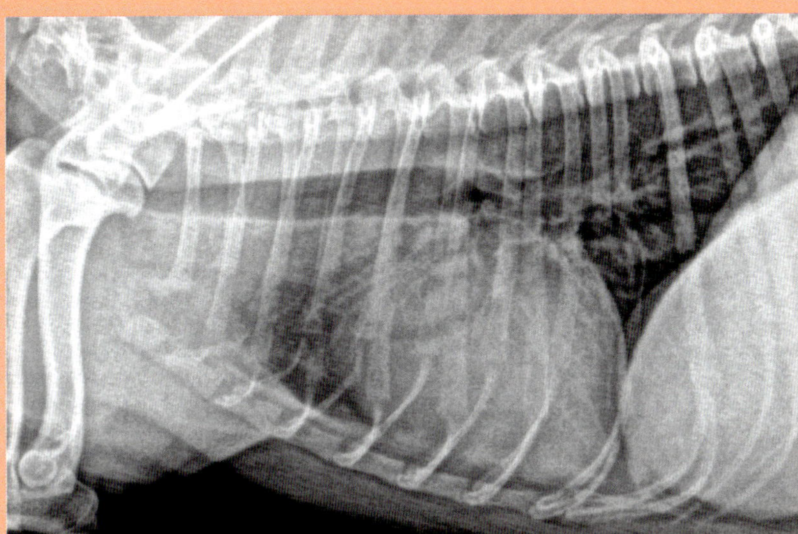

Figure 5. Tracheal collapse and other chronic obstructive respiratory diseases are very common in dogs. Before attributing clinical signs to decompensated congestive heart failure, ensure that the clinical signs are genuinely of cardiac origin.

- Pimobendan, 0.25–0.3 mg/kg orally twice a day.
- An ACEI at the standard dose (e.g. enalapril 0.5 mg/kg orally twice a day); generally, the highest recommended dose range is selected. In well-controlled patients with early, limited clinical signs, a lower dose range can be selected, with dose escalation as the disease progresses.
- Loop diuretics:
  - Furosemide, at a standard dose of 2 mg/kg twice a day. Furosemide dosing is quite variable, and depending on the severity of the pulmonary oedema, it can range from 1 mg/kg twice a day to 6 mg/kg 3 times a day. The current approach is to give the lowest dose at the lowest frequency to maintain the best possible quality of life for the patient.
  - Furosemide can be replaced with torasemide, at a single dose ten times lower than that calculated for furosemide (standard oral dose of 0.2 mg/kg once a day). Torasemide dosing is easier than that of furosemide, which often improves owner compliance with treatment. It is also a good option in patients that have developed resistance to furosemide over time, and its use has not shown to cause greater side effects so far.
- The combination therapy pimobendan + ACEI + furosemide is currently the most common protocol used by cardiologists, but the author prefers to start with a simpler plan in early cases and add drugs as the clinical situation

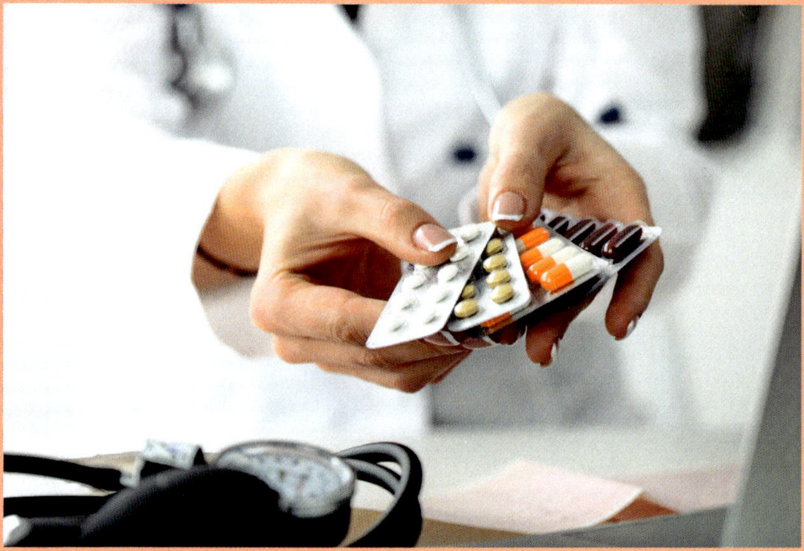

Figure 6. Optimal owner compliance is essential to successful long-term management of CHF.

requires, with the caveat that high-ceiling diuretic monotherapy is not recommended due to the risk of RAAS activation.

- Periodic monitoring of renal function and electrolytes once treatment with diuretics and an ACEI has started, especially in patients with severe CHF and a history of kidney disease or prerenal azotaemia and in cases of long-term aggressive furosemide treatment.
- Spironolactone 0.25–2 mg/kg orally once or twice a day. At this stage, it is typically used as an aldosterone antagonist rather than as a secondary diuretic. The RAA system may be only incompletely blocked with an ACEI, and aldosterone escape may occur; in this case, spironolactone treatment is clearly beneficial. This author recommends the commercial spironolactone + benazepril formulation for simplicity.
- The next ACVIM meeting may bring about a consensus recommendation to add spironolactone to the pimobendan + ACEI + furosemide therapy.
- Digoxin 0.0025–0.005 mg/kg orally twice a day for atrial fibrillation, in order to maintain a plasma concentration of 0.8–1.5 ng/ml (collect a blood sample 8 hours after administration, 7–10 days after starting treatment, and adjust the dose based on digoxin plasma levels) (Fig. 7).
  - Some cardiologists include digoxin even without evidence of supraventricular arrhythmias, but the author does not because it complicates the treatment plan, requires monitoring including plasma digoxin levels and performing ECGs, and lacks evidence that the benefits outweigh the risks of adverse effects.
  - Some cardiologists prefer to give beta-blockers or calcium channel blockers. The author prefers digitalis drugs for this purpose.

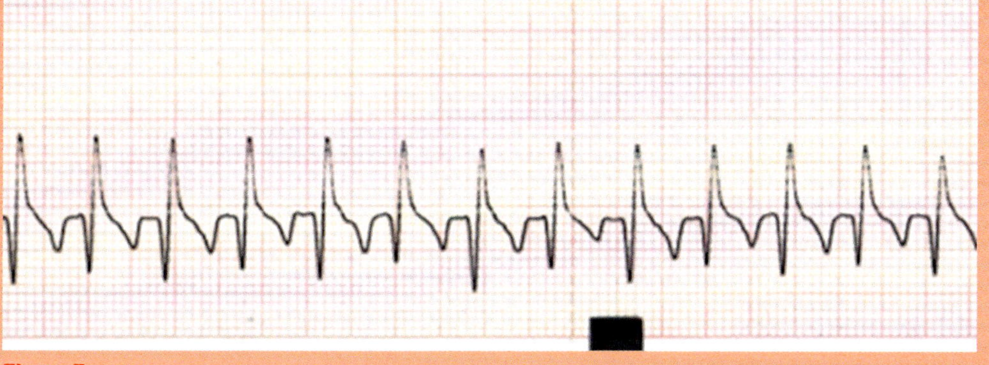

Figure 7. Digitalis remains the treatment of choice for atrial fibrillation and supraventricular arrhythmias.

- Do not give beta-blockers (atenolol, carvedilol, metoprolol), especially without atrial fibrillation, although some clinicians give low doses to stabilised patients. The rationale is that they improve myocardial function and mitigate cardiac remodelling in humans, but no research shows similar effects in dogs. This author does not give them due to the lack of scientific evidence, the need for ECG and blood pressure monitoring, and the risk of adverse effects such as bradycardia, hypotension, and decreased cardiac output.
- Do not give nitroglycerin at this stage.
- Give antitussives and bronchodilators as supportive therapy to mitigate clinical signs, as long as the treatment plan is not overly complex. These measures may help relatively stable patients who also have chronic respiratory disease, a common situation in practice.
- Diet: weight loss from cardiac cachexia is a sign of severe CHF decompensation. It is defined as >7.5 % weight loss relative to the pre-illness weight (without counting any effusions). This is a complicating factor that aggravates the prognosis and is easier to prevent than to treat, so the following are recommended:
  - A palatable balanced diet with adequate caloric content (60 kcal/kg) and low in salt (Fig. 8).
  - Watch for, prevent and combat anorexia.
  - Monitor the patient's weight and evaluate the possible causes of the changes noted.
  - Avoid protein-restricted diets (renal diets), unless concomitant kidney disease exists.
  - Avoid treats, homemade food, and any other high-salt foods.
  - Routine potassium supplementation is unnecessary unless hypokalaemia is detected. Spironolactone and ACEIs are potassium-sparing drugs that counteract potassium loss due to diuretics. Hyperkalaemia is also rare, so high-potassium diets need not be avoided unless blood tests reveal high potassium levels.

- Some cardiologists recommend magnesium supplementation in case of arrhythmias. Supplement only if the electrolyte panel shows hypomagnesaemia.
- Some authors recommend supplementation with omega 3 fatty acids, especially if anorexia, muscle wasting, or arrhythmias occur.

- Perform X-rays and an ECG every six months (sooner if the CHF is not fully stabilised), in addition to monitoring the resting respiratory rate at home.

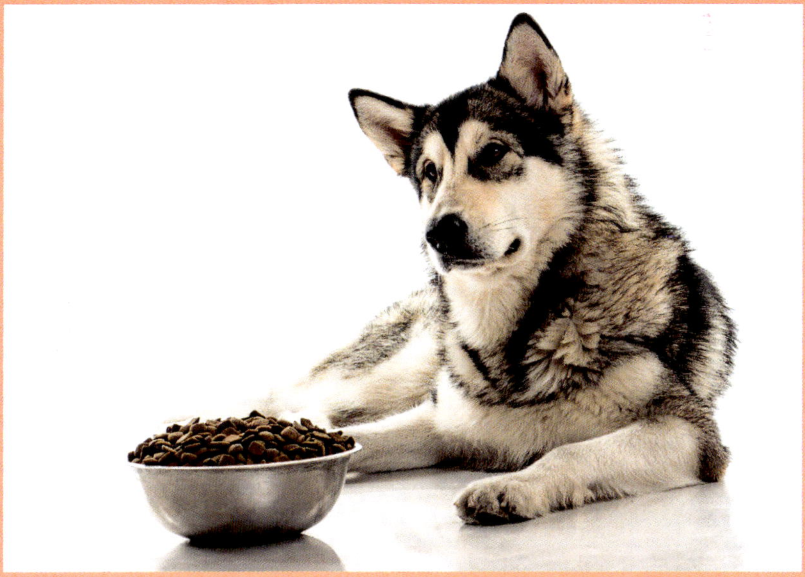

Figure 8. Prevent anorexia with palatable diets with adequate caloric content. Most cardiologists recommend a moderately salt-restricted diet.

OUTPATIENT MANAGEMENT
OF PATIENTS WITH STAGE D CVD-INDUCED CHF

This category includes all patients refractory to treatments given in stage C.

Because CVD is a chronic degenerative disease, conventional treatment eventually becomes insufficient to maintain quality of life, and a more aggressive approach is required.

However, despite the fact that CVD is naturally expected to worsen in all patients, other possible causes of treatment failure include:

- Misdiagnosis of CVD.
- An additional disease (with particular focus on chronic respiratory disease).
- Errors or lack of compliance of owners.

Determine if any of the preceding apply before increasing dosage or adding drugs to the treatment protocol.

Stage D patients do not necessarily require hospitalisation. This section reviews approaches to patients not presenting acutely or severely enough to require hospitalisation.

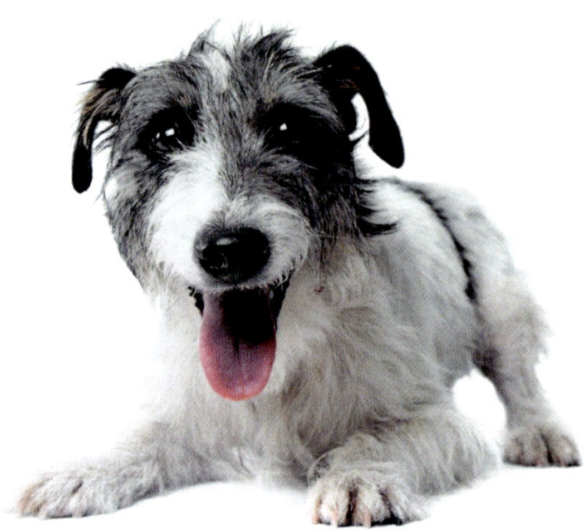

RECOMMENDATIONS

- If the patient is not already receiving triple therapy (pimobendan + ACEI + furosemide), it should be instituted at this time.
- Some authors add a third dose of pimobendan (0.3 mg/kg, 3 times a day).
- Most cardiologists add spironolactone if it is not already being given in order to block aldosterone escape.
- Loop diuretics:
  - Increase the dose and frequency of furosemide as required to reduce pulmonary oedema. Once the situation is controlled, the dose should be lowered to the minimum that allows control of congestive signs (Fig. 9).
  - Torasemide, instead of or in addition to furosemide. Both humans and dogs develop a resistance to furosemide over time when it is given frequently at high doses. Torasemide is an even more potent diuretic than furosemide, and although few studies are available, it can be tremendously useful in this situation. This author has used torasemide for more than twenty years with positive results. Its usage is quite variable: at first, torasemide should be given once a day at a dose one-tenth that of furosemide (for example, replace furosemide 3 mg/kg twice a day with torasemide 0.3 mg once a day). If this fails to control very advanced CHF, the dose may be increased, both drugs may be given (e.g. torasemide 0.3 mg in the morning and furosemide 3 mg/kg at night), or torasemide may be administered twice a day.

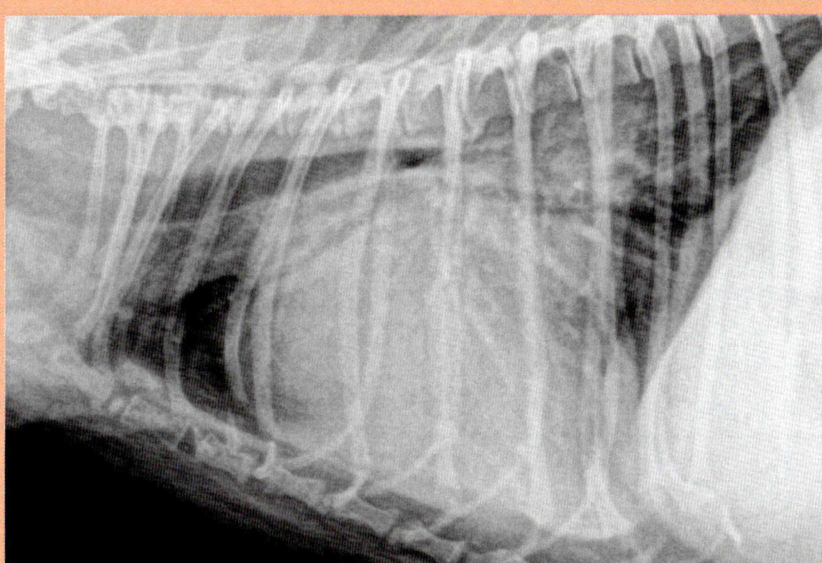

Figure 9. Diuretics are essential to treat pulmonary oedema in dogs with stage D congestive heart failure. An aggressive approach should be taken while monitoring renal function.

- Some authors add thiazides, such as hydrochlorothiazide (e.g. every other day, in addition to furosemide treatment) to bolster furosemide's effect. Acute kidney injury and severe electrolyte disturbances often occur with this treatment, so this author disfavours this strategy in advanced CHF. Torasemide is preferred.
- Monitor renal function and electrolytes 24–48 hours after increasing diuretic dose.

- Digoxin. The remarks on stage C patients apply to those in stage D as well.
- Certain authors give sildenafil (1–2 mg/kg orally twice a day), particularly if pulmonary hypertension is also present.
- Empirically, in refractory terminal cases, the author has successfully given oral nitrates such as isosorbide dinitrate instead of nitroglycerin patches or ointment; the latter formulations are more difficult for owners to handle and thus carry a higher risk of side effects. Since the approval of pimobendan, oral nitrates have fallen into disuse.
- Do not give beta-blockers if the patient is not stable. If they are already being given, decrease the dose to prevent potential complications (hypotension, bradycardia).
- Some doctors give antitussives or bronchodilators as supportive therapy. Keep in mind that bronchodilators are sympathomimetics. If the patient has atrial fibrillation or a very high heart rate, the benefits may not outweigh this adverse effect.
- Diet: all the recommendations for stage C are applicable to this stage. It is critical to avoid excess salt in treats and homemade food.

INPATIENT MANAGEMENT
OF PATIENTS WITH ACUTE CVD-INDUCED CHF

Although the ACVIM guidelines recommend different treatments in stages C and D, this distinction lacks practical significance because patients in both stages are decompensated and at risk of death if corrective measures are not immediately implemented; these measures are nearly the same in both cases.

The acute treatment objectives for these patients focus on the following points:

- Improving preload.
- Improving afterload.
- Decreasing heart rate.
- Improving contractility.
- Decreasing mitral regurgitation.
- Relieving clinical signs associated with low cardiac output and increased venous pressure (preload).

The classic presentation is of an elderly patient with acute pulmonary oedema characterised by severe congestive signs such as exercise intolerance, cough, and dyspnoea at rest, tachycardia, tachypnoea, and sometimes orthopnoea.

Signs of low cardiac output such as weakness, syncope, and hypoxia may also appear.

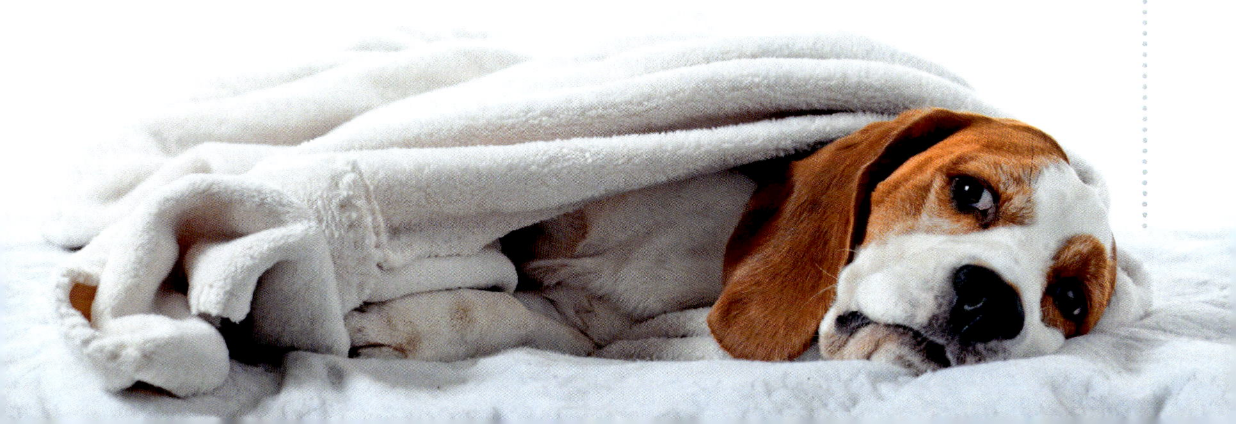

RECOMMENDATIONS

- Place the patient in an oxygen cage or provide nasal or mask oxygen, never stressing the patient. In long-term treatment, manage the temperature and humidity. This is always the first step, even before administering any medication (Fig. 10).
- Place an intravenous line for CRI administration. Do not give fluids.
- Sedate the patient in order to decrease anxiety and tissue oxygen requirements:
  - Butorphanol (0.2–0.25 mg/kg IM/IV) with or without midazolam (0.25 mg/kg).
  - Buprenorphine (0.0075–0.01 mg/kg with acepromazine (0.01–0.03 mg/kg) IV/IM/SC.
- Take thoracic X-rays and avoid forced positioning. If the patient presents with orthopnoea, avoid any stress or manipulation that may compromise ventilation. Take a single lateral view or delay the X-rays until the patient is stable, and give an initial bolus of furosemide (Fig. 11).
- Thoracentesis and paracentesis to ease breathing in patients with pleural effusion or ascites.
- Furosemide:
  - Initial treatment: 1–4 mg/kg IV bolus, depending on the severity of the pulmonary oedema, until the breathing pattern is acceptable. Standard dose: 2 mg/kg. The bolus can be repeated every 30 minutes as needed without exceeding 12 mg/kg total per day.

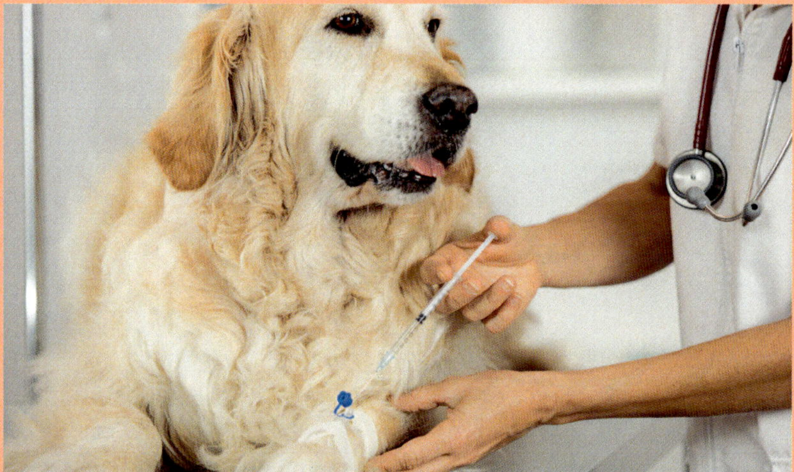

Figure 10. Stabilise the patient with oxygen, place an intravenous line, and sedate the patient prior to any other action such as taking X-rays or starting medical treatment.

- If the patient is critical or the dyspnoea and breathing rate do not improve after 2 hours, give furosemide 1 mg/kg/h as a CRI after at least one initial bolus. Continue the infusion until breathing improves or for a maximum of 4 hours.
- Sodium nitroprusside CRI at a dose of 0.5–1 µg/kg/min for a maximum of 48 hours if pulmonary oedema does not resolve with furosemide.
- Some cardiologists give other vasodilators such as:
  - 2 % Nitroglycerin: approximately 1 cm^3/10 kg for 24–36 hours.
  - Hydralazine: 0.5–2 mg/kg orally.
  - Amlodipine 0.05–0.1 mg/kg orally.
  - All arterial vasodilators should be given with caution. Start with low doses and always monitor renal function, perform an ECG, and check blood pressure. Maintain a systolic blood pressure >85 mmHg or a mean arterial pressure >60 mmHg. Although arterial vasodilators decrease blood pressure, they are recommended in critical patients; by decreasing afterload, they substantially improve cardiac output and potentially maintain blood pressure.

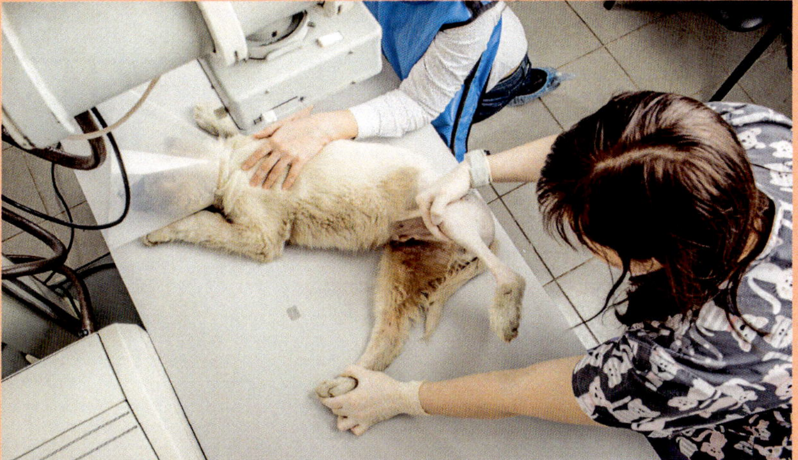

Figure 11. Thoracic X-rays are essential for diagnosing decompensated congestive heart failure and assessing the severity of pulmonary oedema, but the patient must be somewhat stable to avoid danger.

- In cases of hypotension where a fast-acting positive inotrope is necessary, dobutamine can be given as a CRI at 0.5–1 µg/kg/min, re-evaluating every 15–30 minutes, to a maximum of 10 µg/kg/min. Nitroprusside and dobutamine can be given separately or in combination to critical patients for 12–48 hours to improve their haemodynamic status and decrease refractory acute pulmonary oedema.
- Pimobendan 0.3 mg/kg orally twice a day. Some authors recommend adding a third dose. Alternatively, an intravenous formulation can be given.
- An ACEI orally at the standard dose: despite the lack of consensus, most specialists use ACEIs to boost the action of furosemide. Spironolactone can also be started if it is not already in the outpatient protocol.
- Certain authors give sildenafil (1–2 mg/kg orally twice a day), particularly if pulmonary hypertension is also present.
- Give an antiarrhythmic if life-threatening arrhythmias are detected.

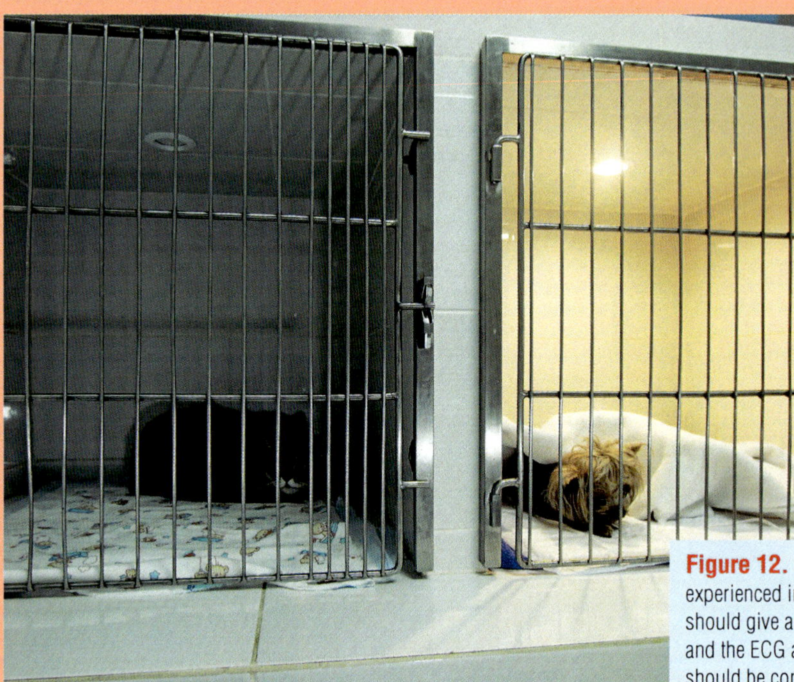

Figure 12. Only clinicians experienced in intensive care should give arterial vasodilators, and the ECG and blood pressure should be continually monitored.

The following diagram summarises the recommended steps (Fig. 13).

Figure 13 FLOW CHART FOR TREATMENT OF A PATIENT WITH CVD AND CLINICAL SIGNS COMPATIBLE WITH DECOMPENSATED CHF

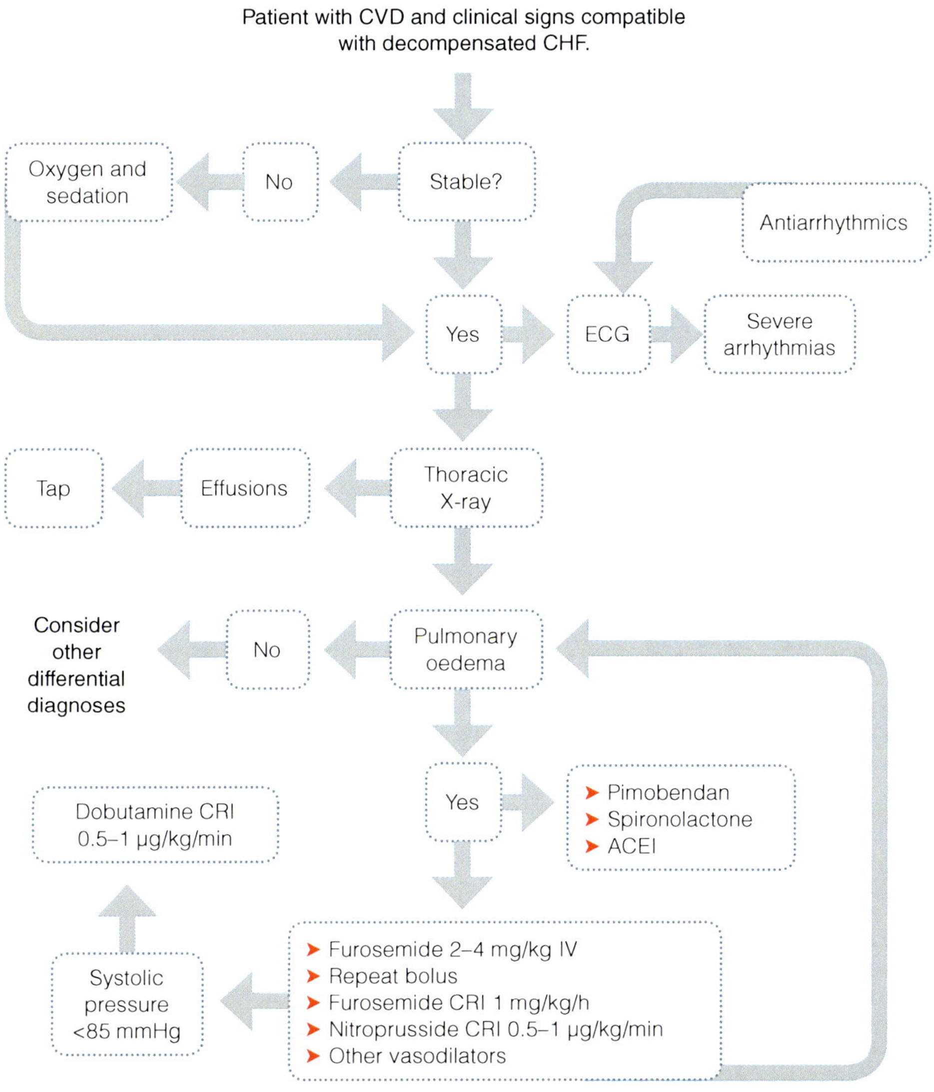

CVD, chronic valvular disease; CHF, congestive heart failure; ACEI, angiotensin-converting enzyme inhibitor.

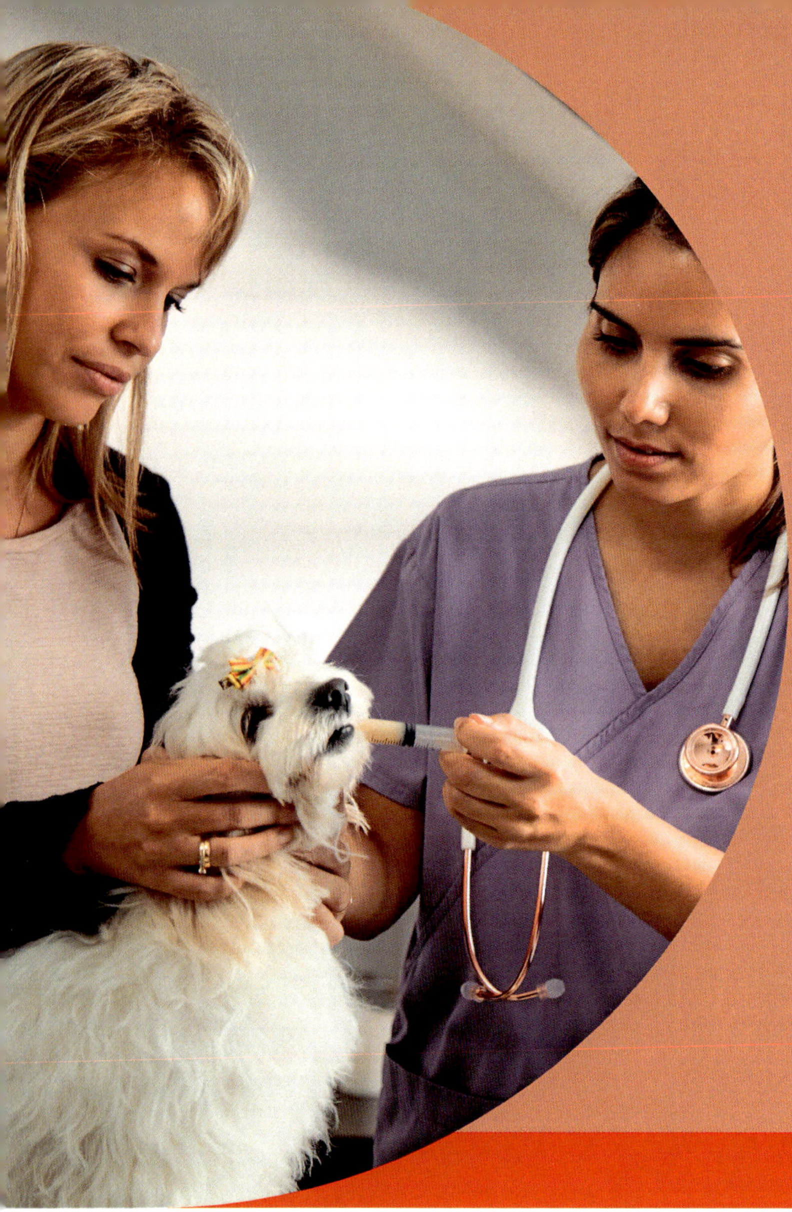

6

CLIENT EDUCATION

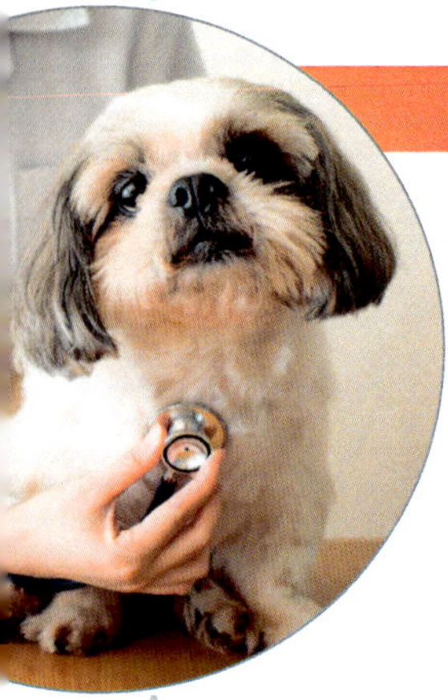

INFORMATION SHEET FOR OWNERS

HOW DOES THE HEART WORK?

The heart is divided into upper chambers called **atria** and lower ones called **ventricles**. It has left and right sides. There are four chambers in total.

The heart is a perfectly synchronised pump: the atria collect the blood and carry it to the ventricles, and the ventricles expel the blood with each heartbeat or cardiac contraction.

CARDIAC FUNCTION

Summary of cardiac cycle:

1. Deoxygenated blood returns from the organs and body systems through the veins to the right atrium.
2. It moves from the right atrium to the right ventricle.
3. With each heartbeat, the right ventricle pumps the blood to the lungs.
4. Oxygenated blood from the lungs collects in the left atrium (LA).
5. It moves from the left atrium to the left ventricle (LV).
6. The left ventricle, which is stronger and more muscular, pumps oxygenated blood throughout the body with each heartbeat.

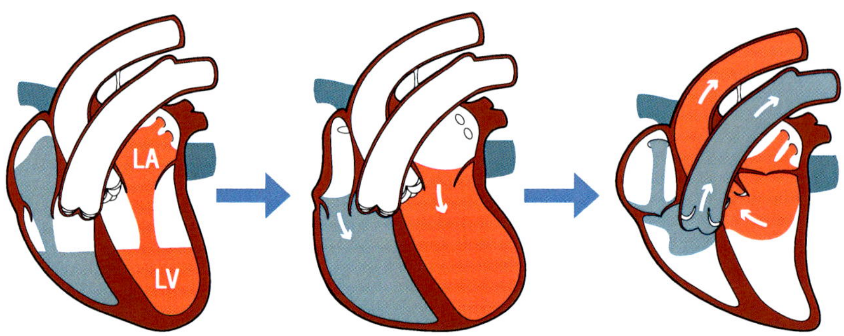

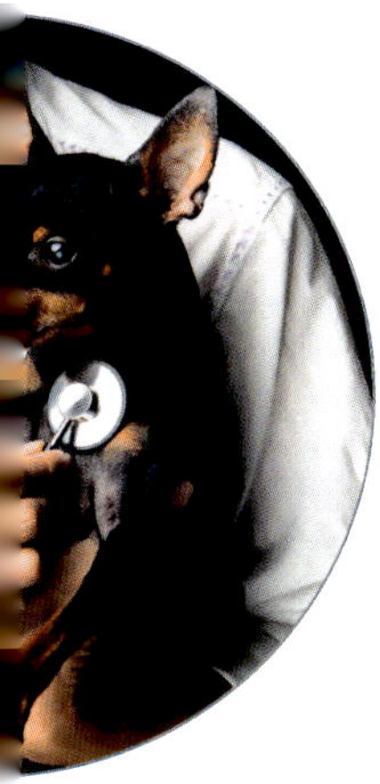

WHAT IS
THE MITRAL VALVE?

The valves must allow or block blood flow correctly at each stage of the cardiac cycle.

The mitral valve regulates blood flow from the left atrium to the left ventricle:

- In point 5 on the previous page, the mitral valve opens to let the ventricle fill with oxygenated blood that the left atrium has collected from the lungs.
- In point 6, the mitral valve closes so that when the left ventricle contracts, the blood does not return to the left atrium and instead spreads throughout the body.

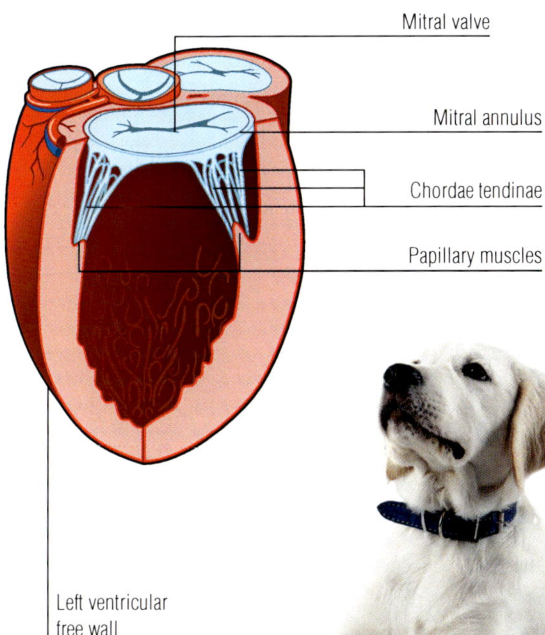

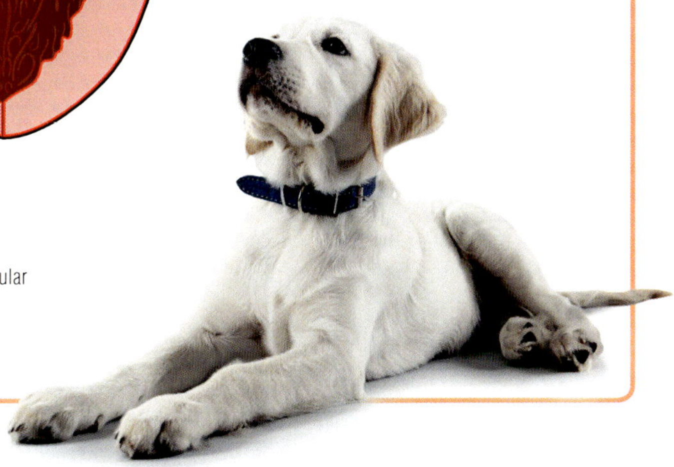

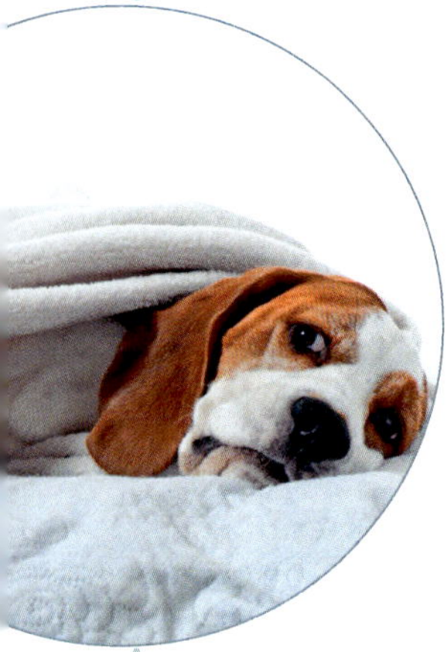

WHAT HAPPENS IF THE MITRAL VALVE DOES NOT CLOSE PROPERLY?

If the mitral valve remains open during ventricular contraction, some blood returns to the left atrium. This has two consequences:

- Less oxygenated blood leaves the heart to travel to the organs and systems.
- Blood refluxes into the left atrium. This is known as **mitral regurgitation**. The left atrium is not as muscular as the ventricle, and it eventually dilates due to the extra volume of blood received with each heartbeat.

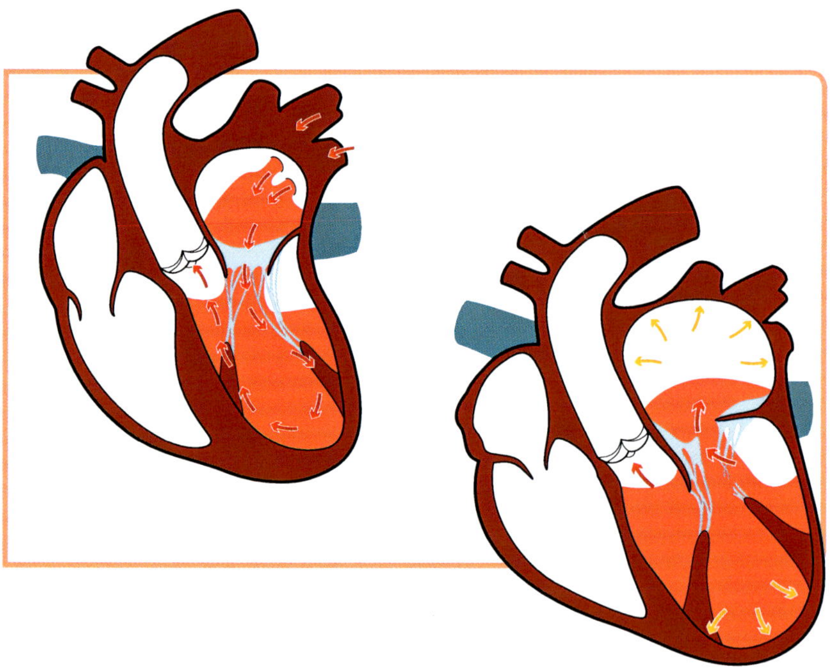

WHAT IS CHRONIC VALVULAR DISEASE

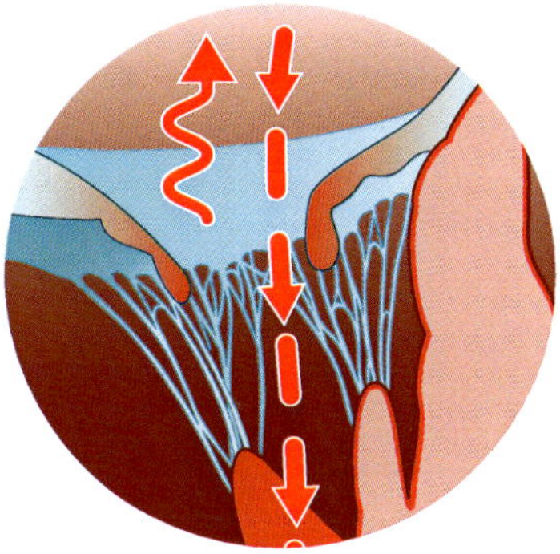

Chronic valvular disease (CVD) is a very common degenerative disease in dogs that affects the mitral valve. The valve eventually becomes deformed and thickens such that it does not fully close, which allows blood regurgitation from the left ventricle with each heartbeat. At the start, the regurgitant volume is low, but it increases progressively as the disease progresses and the valve becomes more affected.

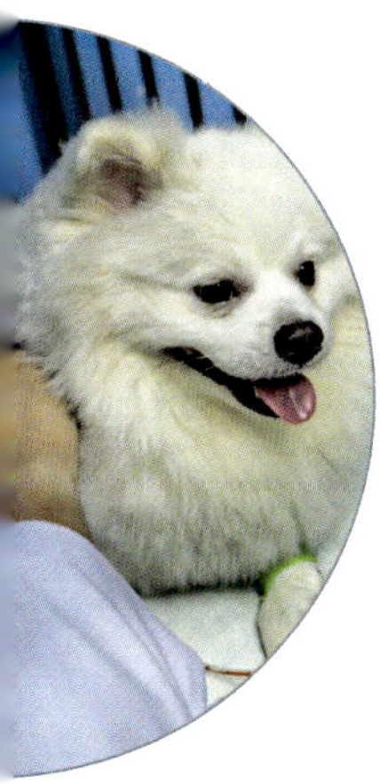

COULD MY DOG HAVE CVD?

The most common heart disease in dogs is chronic valvular disease. It is very prevalent, especially in small elderly dogs.

Statistically, it affects:

- 1 in 3 dogs over 1 year old.
- 1 in 4 dogs over 9 years old.
- 3 in 4 dogs over 16 years old.

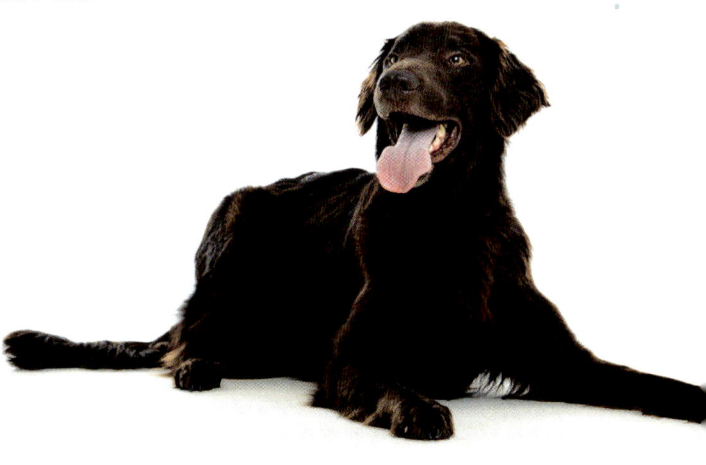

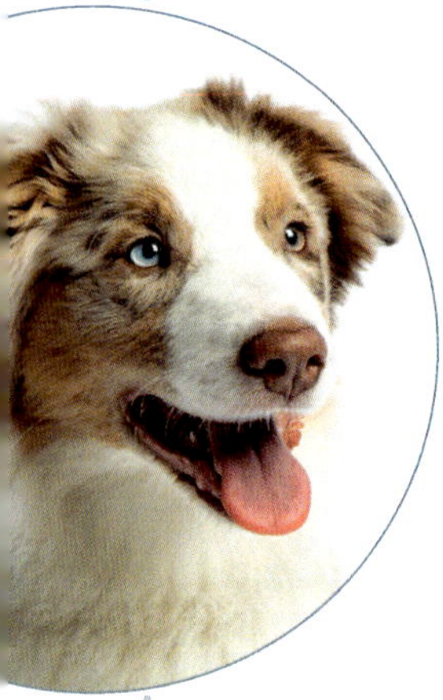

WHAT ARE THE CLINICAL SIGNS OF CVD?

Blood regurgitation into the left atrium produces turbulent flow in the heart, causing a murmur that may be easily detected using a stethoscope.

This murmur is audible as soon as the valve begins to close inadequately, long before left atrial dilation or other signs appear. Later, left atrial dilation and the failure of the compensatory mechanisms cause fluid buildup in the lungs (**pulmonary oedema**), which is responsible for the severe clinical signs that characterise advanced CVD.

Disease stages		Clinical signs in dogs
Stage B1	Subclinical phase in which a murmur is detected, but the heart has not been remodelled.	No clinical signs.
Stage B2	Subclinical period with cardiac remodelling.	No clinical signs.
Stage C or D	Periods in which the heart cannot function adequately and the condition known as congestive heart failure (CHF) develops.	Classic clinical signs such as the following may occur: ➤ Cough. ➤ Respiratory difficulty or increased respiratory rate. ➤ Fatigue during exercise or at rest. ➤ Weight loss. ➤ Abdominal distension. ➤ Episodes of weakness or fainting.

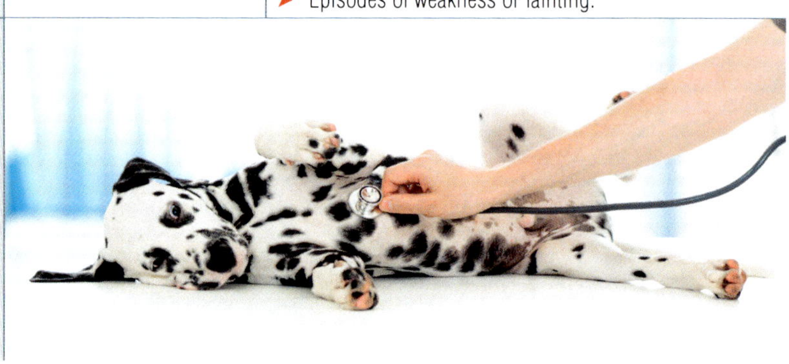

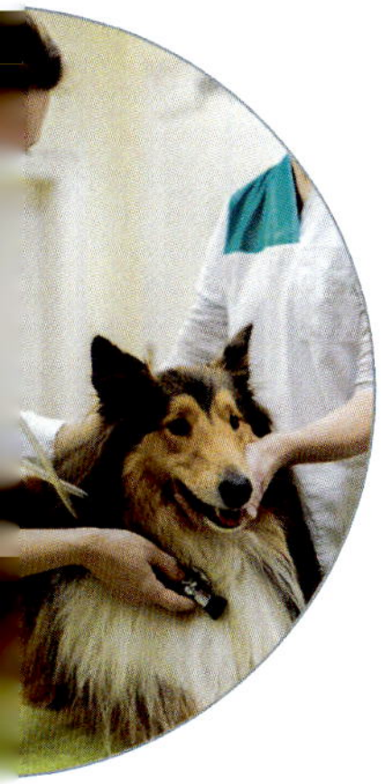

HOW IS CVD DIAGNOSED?

The simple auscultation of a murmur during a routine visit in an adult dog is suggestive of CVD. In this case, other tests such as **thoracic X-rays** and an **ECG** are necessary to detect any changes in the size or silhouette of the heart. X-rays can also reveal pulmonary oedema.

In cases where these tests are inconclusive, an **echocardiogram** may be needed.

IS CVD TREATABLE?

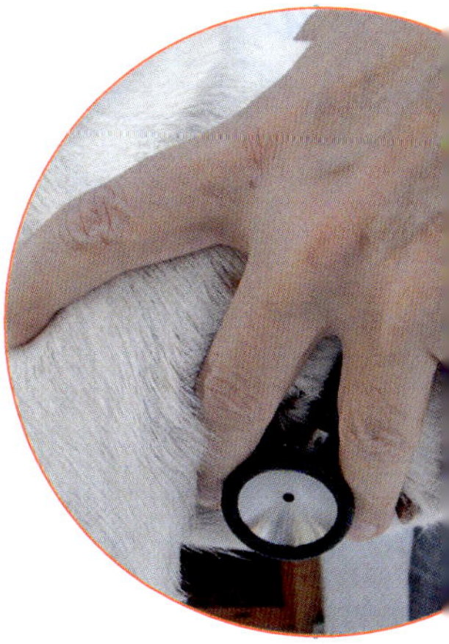

Early detection of the disease and initiation of medical treatment in stage B2 (evidence of changes in cardiac size or silhouette but no clinical signs) can significantly delay disease progression.

Once CHF develops, medications such as **diuretics** and **vasodilators**, are essential to reabsorb fluid from the lungs and ease the burden on the heart. Some cases of advanced CVD require other medications to improve cardiac contractility, decrease the heart rate, and treat cardiac arrhythmias.

These medications extend the life and improve the quality of life of affected dogs.

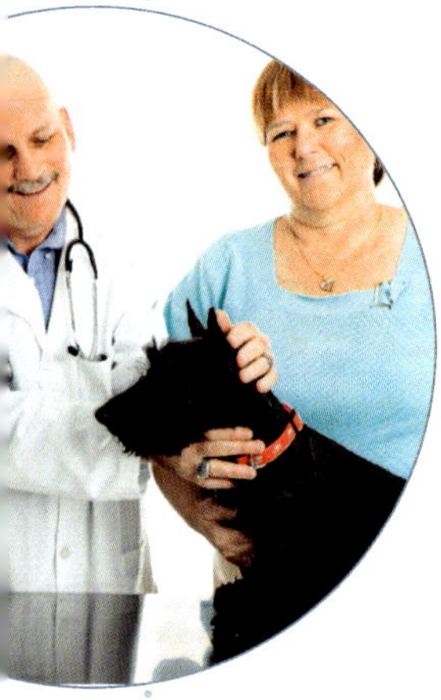

HOW LONG CAN MY DOG LIVE WITH CVD?

This is quite variable, but the disease tends to manifest after age 7 or 8. Many dogs can remain asymptomatic for months or years until they develop CHF, and early treatment in stage B2 extends this time by more than one year on average. In advanced CHF, the treatment significantly prolongs life expectancy and greatly mitigates the signs of the disease.

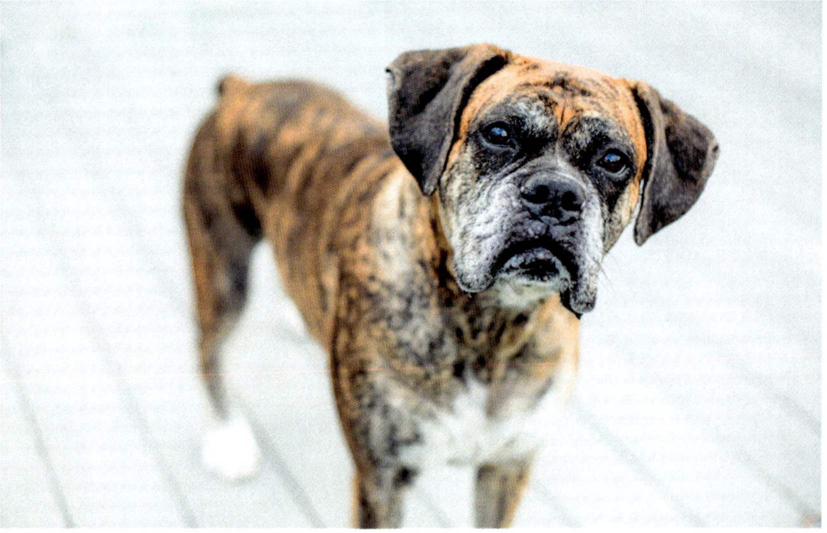

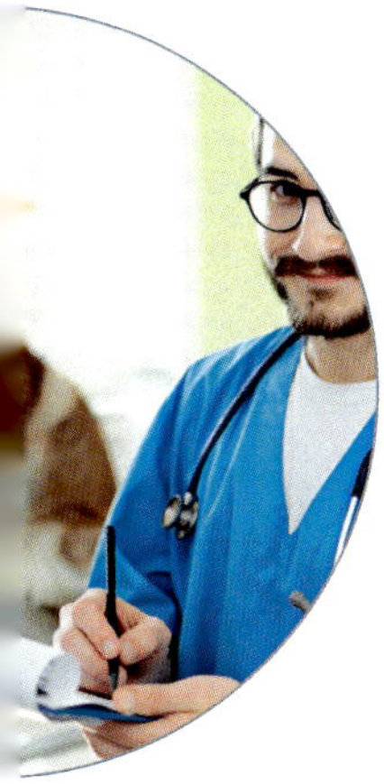

WHAT SHOULD I DO IF MY DOG IS DIAGNOSED WITH CVD?

- Once a murmur is detected, tests are needed to look for changes in the cardiac size and silhouette and to determine if a specific treatment is necessary. If the tests are negative, **regular monitoring** is needed every 6–12 months.
- Once medical treatment is started, **cardiac monitoring** is required every 6–12 months; this should include thoracic X-rays, an ECG, and blood tests to evaluate the cardiovascular status and to prevent possible side effects.
- See your veterinary surgeon if your dog shows clinical signs such as cough, respiratory stress or difficulty, fatigue, weakness, apathy, lack of appetite, fainting, weight loss or abdominal distension.
- Measuring the **resting respiratory rate** at home can be helpful to detect worsening of the disease. A resting or sleeping respiratory rate over 30 breaths per minute for 2 days is sufficient reason to see the vet.
- Providing a **balanced diet** as advised by your veterinary surgeon and avoiding treats and homemade food, which are often high in salt, are crucial to slowing disease progression.
- A dog with CVD can live a relatively normal life.

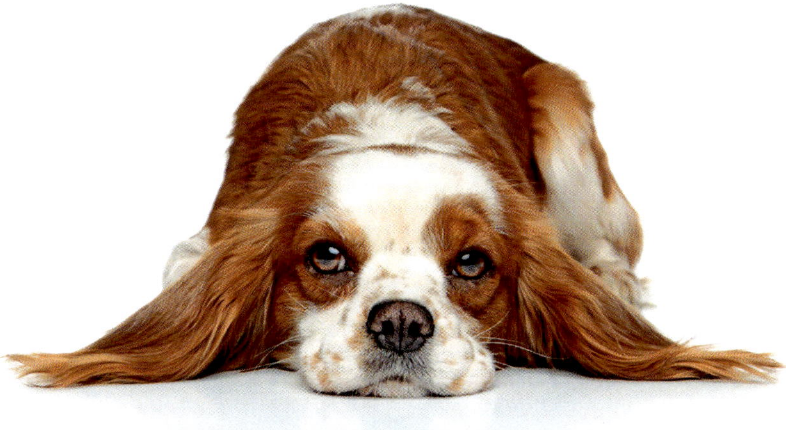

APPENDIX I. TABLE OF DOSES

Active ingredient	Dose	Observations
Furosemide	Outpatient treatment: ➤ 1–2 mg/kg SID, BID, TID, PO Inpatient treatment: ➤ 1–4 mg/kg IV bolus ➤ 1 mg/kg/h IV drip	➤ Increase dose and frequency based on the severity of the pulmonary oedema. ➤ Add in or replace with torasemide in case of refractory pulmonary oedema or if furosemide resistance is suspected. ➤ Monitor renal function and electrolytes.
Torasemide	0.1–0.2 mg/kg SID, PO	As a substitute for furosemide, with the same indications and precautions.
Hydrochlorothiazide	2–4 mg/kg SID, BID, or every other day, PO	➤ Add to loop diuretics for refractory pulmonary oedema. ➤ Risk of kidney disease, electrolyte imbalances, or hyperglycaemia.
Spironolactone	0.25–2 mg/kg SID, BID, PO	As monotherapy or with benazepril.
Pimobendan	0.25–0.3 mg/kg BID, PO 0.1 mg/kg IV	Some authors recommend three doses daily (in stages C and D).
Enalapril	0.5 mg/kg SID, BID, PO	Monitor renal function.
Benazepril	0.25–0.5 mg/kg SID, PO	Monitor renal function.
Ramipril	0.125–0.25 mg/kg SID, PO	Monitor renal function.
Digoxin	0.0025–0.005 mg/kg BID, PO	➤ Ensure its plasma concentration is between 0.8 and 1.5 ng/ml. ➤ ECG monitoring.
Atenolol	0.2–1 mg/kg SID, BID, PO	➤ Start with a half dose. ➤ Monitor renal function, blood pressure, and ECG.
Amlodipine	0.05–0.1 mg/kg SID, PO	➤ Start with a half dose. ➤ Monitor renal function, blood pressure, and ECG.

APPENDIX I. TABLE OF DOSES

Active ingredient	Dose	Observations
2 % nitroglycerin	1 cm^3/10 kg for 24–36 hours	Monitor renal function and blood pressure.
Sodium nitroprusside	0.5–1 µg/kg/min IV drip	➤ Maximum of 48 hours. Can be combined with dobutamine. ➤ Monitor blood pressure.
Isosorbide mononitrate	0.25–0.5 mg/kg SID, PO	
Isosorbide dinitrate	0.25–2 mg/kg/day split into 2–3 doses, PO	
Hydralazine	0.5–2 mg/kg PO	Monitor renal function and blood pressure.
Sildenafil	1–2 mg/kg BID, PO	In case of pulmonary hypertension.
Dobutamine	0.5–1 µg/kg/min IV drip	➤ Reassess every 15–30 min, maximum dose of 10 µg/kg/min. ➤ Monitor blood pressure.

Abbreviations: SID, once daily; BID, twice daily; TID, three times daily; PO, orally; IV, intravenously.

REFERENCES

Adin, DB., Taylor, AW., Hill, RC., et al. Intermittent bolus injection versus continuous infusion of furosemide in normal adult greyhound dogs. *J Vet Intern Med*, 2003; 17:632–636.

Atkins, C., Bonagura, J., Ettinger, P., et al. ACVIM Consensus Statement. Guidelines for the diagnosis and treatment of canine chronic valvular disease. *J Vet Intern Med*, 2009; 23:1142:1150.

Atkins, CE., Keene, BW., Brown, WA., et al. Results of the veterinary enalapril trial to prove reduction in onset of heart failure in dogs chronically treated with enalapril alone for compensated, naturally occurring mitral valve insufficiency. *JAVMA*, 2007; 231:1061–106.

Bernary, F., et al. Efficacy of spironolactone on survival in dogs with naturally-occuring mitral regurgitation caused by myxomatous mitral valve disease. *J Vet Intern Med*, 2010; 24(2):331–34.

Borgarelli, M., Häggström, J. Canine degenerative myxomatous mitral valve disease: Natural history, clinical presentation and therapy. *Vet Clin North Am Small Anim Pract*, 2010; 40:651–663.

Boswood, A., Häggström, J., Gordon, SG., et al. Effect of pimobendan in dogs with preclinical myxomatous mitral valve disease and cardiomegaly: The EPIC Study - A Randomized Clinical Trial. *J Vet Intern Med*, 2016; 30:1765–1779.

Borgarelli, M., Savarino, P, Crosara S., et al. Survival characteristics and prognostic variables of dogs with mitral regurgitation attributable to myxomatous valve disease. *J Vet Intern Med*, 2008; 22:120–128.

Borgarelli, M., Zini, E., D'Agnolo, G., et al. Comparison of primary mitral valve disease in German Shepherd dogs and in small breeds. *J Vet Cardiol*, 2004; 6:27–34.

Buchanan, J.W. Prevalence of cardiovascular disorders. In Fox PR, Sisson, D., Moise, NS. (eds): *Textbook of Canine and Feline Cardiology*, 2nd ed, Philadelphia, 1999, WB Saunders, pp 457–470.

Ettinger, SJ., Benitz, AM., Ericsson, GF., et al. Effects of enalapril maleate on survival of dogs with naturally acquired heart failure. The Long-Term Investigation of Veterinary Enalapril (LIVE) Study Group. *JAVMA*, 1998; 213:1573–1577.

Freeman, LM., Rush, JE., Kehayias, JJ., et al. Nutritional alterations and the effect of fish oil supplementation in dogs with heart failure. *J Vet Intern Med*, 1998; 12:440–448.

REFERENCES

Freeman, LM., Rush, JE., Markwell, PJ. Effects of dietary modification in dogs with early chronic valvular disease. *J Vet Intern Med*, 2006; 20:1116–1126.

Häggström, J., Duelund Pedersen ,H., Kvart, C. New insights into degenerative mitral valve disease in dogs. *Vet Clin North Am Small Anim Pract*, 2004; 34:1209–1226.

Häggström, J., Boswood, A., O'Grady, M., et al. Effect of pimobendan or benazepril hydrochloride on survival times in dogs with congestive heart failure caused by naturally occurring myxomatous mitral valve disease: The QUEST study. *J Vet Intern Med*, 2008; 22:1124–1135.

Hori, Y., Takusagawa, F., Ikadai, H., et al. Effects of oral administration of furosemide and torsemide in healthy dogs. *Am J Vet Res*, 2007; 68(10):1058–1063.

Kvart, C., Häggström, J., Pedersen, HD., et al. Efficacy of enalapril for prevention of congestive heart failure in dogs with myxomatousvalve disease and asymptomatic mitral regurgitation. *J Vet Intern Med*, 2002; 16:80–88.

Lombard, CW., et al. Clinical efficacy of pimobendan versus benazepril for the treatment of acquired atrioventricularvalvular disease in dogs. *J Am Anim Hosp Assoc*, 2006; 42:249–261.

Oyama, MA., Peddle, GD., Reynolds, CA., et al. Use of the loop diuretic torsemide in three dogs with advanced heart failure. *J Vet Cardiol*, 2011; 13(4):287–292.

Peddle, GD., Singletary, GE., et al. Effect of torsemide and furosemide on clinical, laboratory, radiographic and quality of life variables in dogs with heart failure secondary to mitral valve disease. *J Vet Cardiol*, 2012; 14:253–259.

Schneider, M., Bonavaud, S., Ménard, J., Woehrlé, F., et al. Diuretic dose equipotency between torasemide and furosemide in healthy dogs. *Southern European Veterinary Conference*, 2015.

Swenson, L., Häggström, J., Kvart, C., et al. Relationship between parental cardiac status in Cavalier King Charles spaniels and prevalence and severity of chronic valvular disease in offspring. *JAVMA*, 1996; 208:2009–2012.

PHOTOGRAPHY
CREDITS

SHUTERSTOCK.COM

Sanne vd Berg Fotografie: p. IV
Lucky Business: pp. X, 9
ESB Professional: p. 2
WilleeCole Photography: p. 4
135pixels: pp. 5, 14, 23, 100
cynoclub: pp. 8, 64
Dora Zett: pp. 13, 15
wavebreakmedia: p. 16
Victoria Rak: p. 18
Eric Isselee: pp. 18, 20, 35, 110
alexandre17: p. 23
Antonio Gravante: p. 24
Tom Wang: pp. 29, 66
dogboxstudio: p. 31
Billion Photos: pp. 38, 54
Syda Productions: pp. 40, 86
bmf-foto.de: p. 42
Csanad Kiss: p. 46
Lisa A: p. 47
Pressmaster: pp. 49, 113
Di Studio: p. 57
Donna Ellen Coleman: pp. 58, 72
StudioLaMagica: p. 59
JEONGHYEON NOH: pp. 60, 107
AVAVA: p. 63
didesign021: pp. 68, 111
Margarita Arroyave: p. 71
visivastudio: p. 74
alexei_tm: p. 78
DuxX: p. 82
Jagodka: p. 84
BIGANDT.COM: p. 85
IB Photography: p. 87
Andrenko Tatiana: p. 87
Zoriana Zaitseva: p. 89
megaflopp: p. 92
UJ production: p. 95
Csanad Kiss: p. 96
Igor Normann: pp. 99, 108
PRESSLAB: p. 101
Alexpunker: p. 102
Diego Cervo: p. 104
Orawan Pattarawimonchai: p. 106
Africa Studio: p. 107
Dora Zett: p. 109
sommart sombutwanitkul: p. 109
Andrey_Kuzmin: p. 110
InBetweentheBlinks: p. 112
Lisa F. Young: p. 112
Jagodka: p. 113

Published by Servet editorial - Grupo Asís Biomedia S.L.